TRANSPLANT STORY

TRANSPLANT STORY

PHILIP G. THOMAS

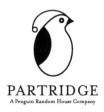

PARTRIDGE

A Penguin Random House Company

To order additional copies of this book, contact
Partridge India
000 800 10062 62
orders.india@partridgepublishing.com

www.partridgepublishing.com/india

CONTENTS

PREFACE

This story is the result of a casual conversation in the doctors' lounge of an operation theater. Conversations between surgeons who are between cases are usually memorable, often hilarious, sometimes instructive, and occasionally productive. Some of the stories they tell are difficult to forget.

Sitting across from me sometime in April this year, Dr. Suresh, Orthopedic surgeon and spine specialist in Lakeshore hospital, Kochi, looked up from his lunch and asked me, "Why don't you write a book on transplant?" Seeing my bewildered expression, he explained that he had written a book on his specialty for the Kerala Bhasha Institute, and they were always on the lookout for educational material. Evidently there is significant public demand for educational literature in Malayalam, and the Literature society is regarded as a reliable and popular source. Consequently, they are in search of such material, and August is when they bring out new books every year.

Mr. Jaikrishnan, on the recommendation of Dr. Suresh, accepted me as a potential author, and assured me that my lack of written Malayalam would be no obstacle as they will translate what I submit in English. To show me what they need, he sent me a recent publication on a medical subject, that soon overwhelmed my halting Malayalam reading abilities. It was a dense treatise that read like a textbook. I found it daunting.

I have no interest in textbooks. Having contributed chapters to some, I have come to the conclusion that these repositories of second hand knowledge are quickly outdated and deservedly dumped every few years with good reason. Former students of mine in India, used to find my attitude incomprehensible. Indians more than anyone else in the world, crave degrees, love textbooks, and have a remarkable ability to memorize them cover to cover. I am reluctant to cater to this weakness or add to their burdens however the case may be perceived. There are however, parts of Transplant Story that might be useful for budding surgeons.

Education is something I find fascinating. I have been involved in teaching medical students and postgraduates in surgery for the last 26 years. In 2009, I got an opportunity to attend the much sought after and oversubscribed course called "Surgeons As Educators" (SAE) conducted by the American College of Surgeons (ACS). The ACS had found that medical doctors in general, and surgeons in particular, are lousy teachers. And this is despite the fact that they do have a certain mastery of their subject, sufficient that one would expect them to be able to teach it. School teachers in comparison often have poor real world experience in what they teach, but their knowledge of good teaching techniques makes up for this deficiency. I realized that like the surgeons who taught me in medical school and during residency, I too was completely ignorant of what is required of an adult educator. I strove thereafter to correct myself, and in time got some recognition for this at the University of Texas where I worked, and also at the American College of Surgeons, where I have been an instructor at the Surgical Education, Principles and Practice (SEPAP) course conducted at the Annual Conference of the College.

The opportunity presented by the Kerala Bhasha Institute to contribute to public education is therefore a golden opportunity. I have, however no experience in educating the general public, who are in no pressing need of what I may have to teach, unlike medical students who are captives of their teachers, boring and incompetent though they might be.

'Needs assessment' is a critical part of adult education. The basic difference between educating children and adults is that the latter only learn what they feel is of practical importance to them. In mulling over the problem and the opportunity presented to me to educate the public about transplant, I decided that a fictional story might serve to create interest and a need to know more, thus enabling me to slip in the educational stuff required.

Transplant is about people healing other people. It is the duty of the medical establishment and society to create the conditions that make this possible. In the context of transplanting organs from deceased individuals, the medical establishment in India has to significantly up their game to international standards before this can become a daily reality. Currently, unfortunately, there is no concerted effort to educate people about organ donation after death in India.

Several studies have shown that the most common reason for refusal by a family when requested to donate organs of their kin after death, is lack of knowledge about transplantation. Reliance on word of mouth is not the best recourse at such a time of intense grief. Studies have also shown that when prior knowledge of transplantation exists, no matter how elementary, consent is often given. Consequently, in countries where cadaver organ transplant systems are established, constant effort is made to keep the public educated about transplantation. This is not happening in India despite 20 years having elapsed since the government enacted the necessary legal and procedural framework for transplantation in India. MOHAN foundation (Multi-Organ Harvesting Aid Network) in Chennai is perhaps the only organization that has focused on education relating to transplant law and ethics, but they have their hands full with a medical establishment that is extremely resistant to change.

People cannot heal other people unless they know what to do (initiative), what to expect (society's response), and what the outcome of their actions is likely to be (competence and transparency in the medical profession).

Transplant professionals in India are in a hurry, and shortcuts have been easy to justify. Live donor transplants continue to be the norm and the numbers of transplants done in India are growing exponentially so that soon India is likely to lead the world in numbers of transplants done. To any observer, however casual, this must appear incongruous. The trauma epidemic probably generates sufficient numbers of organ donors to meet the need for organs in India. Yet we insist, while wasting this precious resource, that our patients find live donors – either coercing family members, or encouraging the organ trade.

Despite having been made illegal in 1994, the trade in organs continues to ensnare recipients and donors with all its avoidable ill effects on individuals and society.

Unlike other countries in Asia, even the more economically advanced ones, common people in India have no entrenched opposition to organ donation after death. This was amply demonstrated 20 years ago when a small group of like minded individuals in Bangalore started cadaver organ retrieval and allocation on the same lines as the US, and surprised everyone by being successful. Their organization called Foundation for Organ Retrieval and Transplant Education (FORTE) was dissolved when the state government set up an organization called ZCCK (Zonal coordination committee, Karnataka) to coordinate cadaver organ donation and transplantation in Karnataka.

Similar organizations were created by the governments of Maharashtra and Tamilnadu. The latter has become a beacon to the rest of India. Determined to remove obstacles to implementation of the Transplant Act, Dr. Amalorpavanathan, a Vascular surgeon, not himself involved in transplant, and Dr. Davidar, an IAS officer with a PhD, started working on the problem and by 2005 had formulated the most detailed set of rules that has ever accompanied a law anywhere in India. To quote Dr. Davidar, this is the only example of a statute that actually sets forth algorithms and spells out in detail the steps of procedure to implement the law in letter and spirit. Between them, and MOHAN foundation, they jump started cadaver organ transplant in the state. Today, Tamil Nadu leads India in the science and practice of transplantation notching up successes in liver, heart, and lung transplantation.

It would be fair to say that if you need a heart, lung or liver transplant today you would be better off living in Chennai than in Hong Kong, Beijing, Seoul, or Tokyo. So profound is the impact of altruism on progress.

The most recent entrant in this field of governmental involvement in deceased donor organ transplantation, is KNOS, the Kerala Network of Organ Sharing.

Set up in 2012 under the Government of Kerala, and widely acknowledged to be the brainchild of Dr.Ramdas Pisharody, Dean of Trivandrum Medical College, and a Kidney transplant specialist himself, KNOS has done surprisingly well.

The dual name of the organization – KNOS Mrithasanjeevani – was itself a masterstroke combining Sanskrit and English, ancient and modern. The name broadcast and linked its mission with UNOS, the apical transplant organization in USA which sets standards worldwide, and the legend of Hanuman who rushed to the Himalayas to find and bring back a life restoring efflorescence for Lord Ram and his brother Laxman who lay dying in a battlefield in what geographically is today the state of Kerala.

Kerala is unique in many ways. With health statistics to equal any developed country, a strong political movement of communism, little or no religious fundamentalism, bigotry or terrorism, and 100% literacy, this strip of lush tropical greenery between the Arabian Sea and the geologically ancient mountain range called the Western Ghats has always cooked up its own exclusive social flavors.

In the context of transplantation, Kerala's distinctive essence has been the unprecedented frequency with which organ donation has been initiated by families of brain dead individuals. Next of kin, seeing for themselves that their patient appears to have no hope of survival from some primary neurological insult or injury, are known to initiate the discussion about organ donation, and have pressurized lackadaisical Neurosurgeons and physicians to facilitate retrieval of whatever organs are transplantable.

Working night and day without any remuneration, other than being on the payroll as Nephrologist at Medical College, Trivandrum, is Dr.Noble Gracious, Nodal Officer of KNOS. True to his name, with gentle demeanor, he has been continuously on call since KNOS was founded, clarifying legal and procedural doubts and settling inane arguments related to Brain Death testing, certification, medicolegal cases, and expenses. He has, in the middle of the night, obtained government recognition of hospitals where a potential donor was located; and empanelled specialists to give permission for organ retrieval. With his crew of three coordinators, they allocate organs, do community outreach and education, liase with government, police and medical specialty organizations, and for the first time ever in India, have started tracking transplant outcomes.

Like conversations in the Operation Theater, I hope that this story will be memorable, and instructive. If Transplant Story helps increase the level of awareness and serves to educate the public in Kerala and perhaps the rest of India, if it can build on the work of individuals like Noble and Ramdas, I will have proved myself worthy to call myself their friend, a man who returned to his ancestral home and put his shoulder to the wheel of the chariot they have so valiantly been driving forward.

Readers might believe they recognize some of the individuals portrayed or caricatured in this story. Adherence to real experience is necessary if fiction is to serve its purpose of revealing truth. I am reluctant to throw out the usual disclaimer that this story 'bears no resemblance' to real characters and incidents. I would like, rather, to quote Arundhati Roy, who when questioned about her famous story describing attitudes and social pathology in Kerala, answered an interviewer with the memorable line: "the starting blocks are real, but the run is pure fiction".

Dedicated to all those who work behind the scenes, by day and by night, to make transplantation of organs from deceased donors possible. Coordinators, hospital administrators, nurses, social workers, police officers, roadside rescue ambulance personnel, pilots and drivers. You will find them in these pages. They make it possible for people to heal other people. They save lives of patients they do not know, and with whom they have no direct connection. They are the mark of societies that have embraced the highest ideals of modern science and altruism.

And to my wife, Rebecca, who served and led FORTE (Foundation for Organ Retrieval and Transplant Education), a small group of like-minded individuals who succeeded twenty years ago in getting neurosurgeons, transplant surgeons and forensic specialists to work together; trained ICU counselors to obtain consent for organ donation after death from families who had never heard of it before; and achieved successful retrieval, allocation, and sharing of organs between hospitals and across states for the first time in India.

PART I

THE DIAGNOSIS

When asked the secret of his success, Mohammed Aliyar Kunju, Kunju to his friends, liked to say it was because of a vow he made early in life that he would owe no man anything. His wife, Ayesha, who was not so free with secrets, once tried to dissuade him from giving his recipe away so readily by saying some people might think what he really meant was that he always gave as good as he got. To which Kunju, who had once been a contender for the light heavyweight spot on the national boxing team, laughed and said he was fine with such misunderstanding.

It was, therefore, not a comfortable feeling for this boxer-turned-businessman to have to wonder at the age of 57 to whom he now owed his life.

Disaster had struck with no prior warning. Kunju was in the back seat of his car being driven to work. He liked to read the newspaper and not pay attention to the hypercompetitiveness of his fellow citizens swirling around the car in an assortment of scooters, motorcycles, autorickshaws, cars and buses. It was just another day, another typical morning rush hour in Kochi.

When he saw the spreading blood stain on the newspaper it was a moment before he realized where it had come from. He had burped to relieve what he thought was dyspepsia from the heavy dinner of the night before when he was hosting his overseas clients, and without warning bright red blood had erupted from his mouth and landed on the Politics page. The election news which had so absorbed his interest faded as he looked around, confused as to where the blood had come from. Then another gush of vomit followed the first, this time shooting over the top of the front seat, some of it rebounding from the back of the headrest onto his starched white shirt front while the rest flowed over and onto the floor mats in front. In a dreamlike sequence he heard Mustafa his trusted driver yelping with fear and hitting the horn. Blaring the horn was Mustafa's incurable reaction to anything happening on the road. He remembered thinking he would have to lecture Mustafa again about this. Then he saw Ayesha. He told her "Don't worry", as he swayed onto his side on the back seat, and everything went dark.

"Variceal bleeding. Cirrhosis liver. Type II diabetes. Obesity."

These were the words written under Diagnosis on his discharge summary when he was ready to get out of hospital a week later.

The diabetes he had known about. Never having had much interest in the workings of the human body, it was, as far as he was concerned, more Ayesha's problem than his. She kept track of his pills and he swallowed them dutifully more due to her insistence, than because he thought they did him any good.

But obesity? Where had that come from? He had 'nalla vannam' the good fat, the unmistakable sign of prosperity distributed with dignity around his middle. And they called it a disease? He wanted to object. Nobody could call him fat, even if it were true.

"Forget it", was Ayesha's response to his objections.

She was more concerned about the diagnosis of cirrhosis liver.

"This is a disease of drunkards. How can they say you have this disease? What will people say?" Ayesha sounded indignant.

"Who cares what they think. Why would anyone know anyway? I am feeling fine now." Kunju said placatingly.

"What do you mean, 'how would anyone know?' Your brother's wife has been very interested in everything. She has been listening to everything the doctors say. They were asking me if you drink alcohol. All kinds of personal questions! It seems they sent your blood to test for alcohol when you arrived! The nurse told me the result, that's how I found out!"

"What was the result?" Kunju asked mildly

"Of course it was negative. I told them they could have asked before secretly doing the test. We are devout Muslims!"

"It was not done secretly. I was unconscious when Mustafa brought me here."

"I am fed up with Mustafa also!" Ayesha was not in a mood to be placated.

"Why?" asked Kunju "I probably owe my life to him for racing through traffic to bring me to the hospital. I am glad I don't remember any of it! I must give him some reward. He had asked me for a loan of fifty thousand. I think I will just give it to him."

"You will do nothing of the kind! He is going around telling everybody the story. Very dramatic! He says you told him 'Don't worry' before you became unconscious!"

Kunju stared at her silently. Ayesha recognized the intense look he would get when he had to tell her something really important.

"He is right, I did say that, Ayesha," Kunju said quietly, "but it was not to him. It was to you. I saw your face like you were there in the car beside me. I felt it was the last moment of my life, and I wanted to tell you not to worry."

There is a medical term for what Kunju described: 'near death experience'.

The diagnosis of 'variceal bleeding' was made soon after he arrived in the Emergency Room unconscious and covered with blood that he had vomited in the car. His blood pressure was low.

"Eighty by palp," the nurse who received him called out.

Shortly after they called a "Code blue" on him as his breathing slowed, and his pulse became impalpable.

Like a herd of rampaging buffalo the code team and all nurses and doctors in the vicinity of the Emergency Room rushed in to resuscitate the new arrival.

Somebody slapped EKG leads on him and recorded the heart rate going slower and slower.

"Atropine!" was called out.

"No response!" Then, "He is fibrillating!" as the monitor recorded the regular pattern disappearing to be replaced by a wavy, squiggly line.

"Start massage! Get ready to shock him!" yelled the anesthetist who was leading the code team. A burly male nurse started cardiac massage. Another nurse dragged the defibrillator to the bedside.

"Jelly! I need some more jelly!" she called, applying what she had to the electroshock paddles.

The paddles were applied to his chest.

"Stand clear everybody!"

Wham! The first shock barely made Kunju's shoulders twitch. The squiggly line continued unchanged on the heart monitor.

The defibrillator whined as they cranked it up to the next power setting.

Wham! This time the shock lifted Kunju almost off the bed.

"Normal tracing!" The Anesthetist sounded relieved and triumphant at the same time. "OK, stop the massage, and get ready to intubate! I want an NG tube placed, and I want a central line. Large bore peripheral iv and start normal saline. Five hundred ml bolus! A full set of labs and type cross 4 units blood!"

Orders were fired fast and furiously, as Kunju was prepared to be shifted on a ventilator to the endoscopy room for emergency upper GI endoscopy. The bright red blood vomited earlier and the same coming out of the tube placed in his stomach indicated the source of bleeding to be in his esophagus or stomach.

The gastroenterologist was waiting gowned, gloved, and with protective goggles as Kunju was rolled in and transferred from his trolley to the endoscopy table. When the anesthetist gave the green signal, the endoscopy was begun and the source of bleeding found to be large tortuous veins in the esophagus, one of which had just popped and was gushing blood. (see a live video of endoscopy and banding of a bleeding varix on *www. organtransplantinformation.com*)

Expertly snagging the bleeding point on the vein, the gastroenterologist slipped an occlusive band onto the vein effectively strangling the flow of blood to the puncture point.

The crisis now averted, and the anesthetist happy, the gastroenterologist proceeded to complete his examination of the esophagus and the stomach. What he saw worried him. The 'varices' – large dilated and tortuous veins were to be seen not only in the esophagus, but lower down in the stomach as well.

Varices in the stomach are harder to control and tend to bleed more torrentially than their cousins in the esophagus above. In the past, surgery to tie off the bleeding veins and control hemorrhage was the only answer to bleeding varices in the stomach. In the esophagus they could be controlled more easily through the endoscope with much less risk of life-threatening complications.

It was only a matter of time before the bleeding would recur.

No telling when, or where.

With the crisis averted, the Gastroenterologist could begin the "work up". It is not enough to diagnose varices, the cause – usually in the liver - needs further evaluation.

A battery of blood tests including Liver function tests and ultrasound scan of the liver were done, while Kunju was still unconscious in the ICU. A couple of days after he awoke and was transferred back to the regular room, a CT scan of the abdomen was also performed.

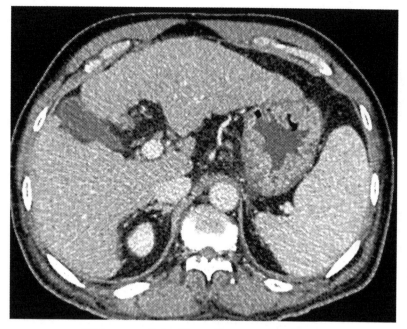

CT scan of the liver showing cirrhosis

Fig 1 (page 10): CT scan of the liver showing cirrhosis. The liver is on the right side (left side of the picture). On the opposite side is the stomach. It appears dark grey which is fluid in the stomach, with one area of black which is the appearance of swallowed air in the stomach. The spleen is the structure behind the stomach. It is larger than normal when the liver has cirrhosis.

The outline of the liver is not smooth. The presence of nodules and bumps are clearly seen. Around the liver is fluid, called ascites which separates it from the bones and muscles of the abdominal wall. (Picture courtesy Dr. Rajesh Antony, Lakeshore Hospital, Kochi, Kerala)

Ayesha was more interested in seeing the scan pictures than Kunju, and would ply the doctors and nurses with dozens of questions.

"They will get irritated with you if you ask so many questions," Kunju was concerned.

"Don't worry. I know who to ask and who not to ask," came the reply.

Indeed Ayesha with her ready smile and charming ways had already established Kunju as the VIP patient on the unit. It was clear to all the nurses and doctors who the 'go-to' person was when it came to the care of their most serious patient. As is typical in Indian hospitals where patients pay their own bills, and every expensive item has to be paid for before it can be used, the quality of care could depend a lot on who was at the bedside with the patient. Ayesha handled the payments and saved all receipts in a folder. Test results and scan reports went in another folder. Mustafa waited downstairs in the lobby, his cell phone at the ready, running errands and taking Ayesha home and back when needed.

The whole family had gone into crisis mode. Their children Raza and Shehnaz who were studying in colleges in other states came home, and were made responsible for crowd control. Friends and family who rushed to the hospital the moment they heard the news were met downstairs in the lobby by Raza or Shehnaz and given an update, then Mustafa would bring them up to the room briefly, and herd them out as soon as they had paid their respects.

The medical and nursing staff looking after Kunju could not help but be impressed by the way his immediate family rallied around and conducted themselves. But it was clear that the person in charge was Mom.

And so it was to Ayesha that the doctors first mentioned that they would be referring Kunju to a Transplant center.

He needed to be evaluated for a liver transplant.

Ayesha's first reaction to this unexpected news was to conceal it from Kunju and everyone else as well. The second reaction was to take him to another hospital and get a second opinion.

After mulling it over for a few hours, she realized that the two were mutually exclusive. She would not be able to suggest going to another hospital without Kunju and everyone else wanting to know why. And that would be the end to concealment. She decided to tell the children first. Shehnaz had already figured out that behind the cheerful exterior, her mother was a very worried woman.

"We need to know what is going on, Mom," Shehnaz insisted, "Raza and I are adults now."

The conference with the kids went much better than Ayesha could have anticipated. She barely said the words 'liver transplant' and Raza had his smart phone out googling the condition. Ayesha was much more tolerant than Kunju to the kids playing with their smart phones while their parents spoke to them. Shehnaz crowded in with her brother looking over his shoulder as he searched the internet.

"Keep talking, Mom", she said not taking her eyes off the screen, "we're listening."

What the children found out on the internet was frightening, and oddly reassuring at the same time. First they searched "cirrhosis", and Ayesha was glad to learn that alcoholics were not the only ones affected. Alcohol was often implicated in cirrhosis, but often only as an accessory agent to some other underlying condition. In the west and in affluent communities worldwide, obesity with associated fatty liver disease was often the underlying condition resulting in progressive liver injury, resulting in cirrhosis. This was particularly true for people who also had diabetes. There was now a newly minted term - "metabolic syndrome" in which multiple organ systems were affected as a consequence of obesity.

When Kunju heard the research on his illness, he remembered his 'fighting weight' of 76 kg when he was 19 years old. In his forties he had weighed in at 104 kg. Since being diagnosed with diabetes, he had lost some weight, and now fluctuated between 92 and 98 kg. Some days he had noticed his feet would be swollen, but he thought it was due to being on his feet all day. When he woke up in the mornings it was usually gone.

The matter of seeking a second opinion without the whole neighborhood finding out was resolved when Raza and Shehnaz photocopied all his records, and sent them as email attachments to a doctor in the US who was a good friend of Ayesha's brother who lived in New York.

The very next day, Ayesha's brother called confirming that the doctors he had consulted in New York had looked at his reports and agreed that he needed to be evaluated as soon as possible for a liver transplant.

Raza had him on Skype so the whole family could see their New York relative while he spoke. He looked worried, and kept glancing at Ayesha.

"I am sure they have good transplant specialists there, Uncle, can we bring him to New York for the transplant?" asked Shehnaz

"That's a good question, Shehnaz," came the voice over the internet, switching from Malayalam to American accented English, as her Uncle once again looked worriedly at her mother, 'and it was in fact the first question I asked the specialists here. Unfortunately the rules and policies governing Transplant are very different from any other kind of medical treatment. They do not allow foreigners to come here for a transplant."

"Why is that?" asked Raza, "is it because we are Muslims?"

"No Raza, that is not the reason. The reason is that organs like the liver are freely gifted to society by the family members of someone who has died, and the government has to guarantee that they are given to someone who is also of this society. I am told that this policy is not peculiar to the US. It is true of all countries. In fact even in India a foreigner cannot come to a Transplant center and get a heart or liver transplant donated by a deceased donor. So trying to get his transplant operation in India is the only hope. I am sorry. I am afraid I can't be of much more help."

Raza was not satisfied with his American uncle's answer, and immediately dived back into the internet search engines he was familiar with. Slowly he put together the facts.

Liver transplantation had been started in America in the 1960s. Initial attempts failed, and after a moratorium of a few years during which techniques were refined in the lab, success was achieved in the 1970s due to the work of Dr. Tom Starzl, the pioneer in the field. It was only in 1983 that the National Institutes of Health in America declared that liver transplantation was no longer an "experimental procedure" and this opened up the treatment to be widely applied. Soon, insurance companies began paying for the operation, and in countries in Europe and in Australia where health care was government funded, hospitals began doing liver transplantation.

The donors were all "deceased donors". In other words these donors were individuals who had suffered "brain death".

The recognition of brain death followed the development of Intensive Care in modern medicine. Intensive Care units were developed all around the world. These units catered to patients who needed intensive monitoring using increasingly complex electronics to continuously check the working of heart and lungs by monitoring heart rate and rhythm, blood oxygenation, and the functioning of other vital organs like the kidneys which depended on a good blood pressure and oxygen delivery. During and after World War 2, blood transfusion, antibiotics and dialysis had become widely available, and the skill required to manage patients needing these treatments were developed all over the world.

Suddenly it became possible to save patients with heart and kidney and liver failure who once would enter a familiar downward spiral of multi-organ failure and quickly die.

Catastrophic brain injury, however, represented a peculiar problem. These patients suffered from severe brain swelling following injury, or stroke, and because skull bones create a confined space the swelling would squeeze the blood supply in the brain to a point where it would cease altogether. Even as Neurosurgeons developed the skills to save many of these unfortunate patients, it became clear that in some, neurological injury was not reversible. Many of these patients had functioning kidneys, liver and heart when they were admitted to the Intensive Care Unit, and when brain death occurred, gradually all these organs would also fail. It became necessary to recognize this situation early in order to conserve scarce resources, and properly counsel grieving family members to better manage their grief and avoid conflicts or suspicions of medical error. In 1962, Harvard University developed the system of diagnosing brain death at the bedside, and these became known as the Harvard Criteria. In later years as medical science and particularly advances in imaging took place with the development of CT, MRI and Nuclear Medicine scans, the Harvard Criteria became more and not less relevant. The set of simple bedside tests described in the 1960s consistently diagnosed complete cessation of blood circulation within the brain.

What was being called 'brain death' is effectively brain gangrene due to the loss of blood supply to the brain. Concealed by the bones of the skull, and protected from secondary bacterial infections that give exposed gangrenous tissue their characteristic putrid odor, brain gangrene – the official term is liquefaction necrosis – is nevertheless as fatal as gangrene anywhere else. In fact, for obvious reasons, much more so.

Meanwhile, so skilled had ICU doctors and nurses become in preserving function in vital organs like the heart, lungs and kidneys that it was realized that, if you were to move fast, these organs could be transplanted to save the lives of people with end stage organ failure.

The concept of brain death was difficult for some societies to accept. In many countries where Intensive Care facilities were poor or non-existent, no doctor ever diagnosed brain death or felt the need to do so. This was the situation in India till the 1990s when opening up of the bureaucratic socialized economy had resulted in a major expansion of medical services in the private sector. Gone were the days of patients suffering at the mercy of '*baboos*' running government hospitals, and making decisions as to who got proper medical care, and which hospital got what equipment. The most significant change seen in India was the increase in the number of ICU beds available all over the country with all the advanced medical monitoring equipment and ventilators regarded as "state-of-the-art" all over the world.

The legislature at the center and in the states had adopted the Human Organs Transplant Act in India in 1994. This statute had propelled India into the ranks of the most advanced countries as far as Transplant science is concerned. The law recognized Brain Death, and permitted gifting of organs by the next-of-kin of a deceased individual to anyone in need of a transplant. Subsequent modifications of the Act permitted retrieving of transplantable organs from any hospital where a potential donor was located and expanded the lists of doctors and medical specialists who could certify the death for purposes of organ donation.

In Kerala, the state government had, under the leadership of Dr. Ramdas Pisharody, Dean of Trivandrum Medical College, and a leading nephrologist of national and international repute, established the Kerala Network of Organ Sharing in 2012, also called "Mrithasanjeevani".

Meanwhile, a few high profile organ donations took place with Fr. Davis Chiramel, a catholic priest, and Mr. Ouseph Chittilapilly, a prominent businessman and philanthropist, donating their kidneys to persons in need. A movie producer scored a box office hit with "Traffic" - the story of a race against time on the congested roads of Kerala with a transplant team racing against time, and an antiquated system of roads and traffic management, to get a heart from the hospital where the donation took place to the Transplant center.

The most widely read Malayalam newspaper in the world, Malayala Manorama began profiling the stories of deceased organ donors and the recipients whose lives they saved. The Kerala government, starting in 2013, held a function honoring deceased donors with a plaque and public recognition of their families at a glamorous and well publicized function in a former palace of the Trivandrum royal family.

A tipping point was reached. Suddenly, the highly literate society of Kerala, addicted to their morning newspapers, and always interested in whatever was new in medical science, was sensitized to the issue and organ donations took off. Hospital Administrators and Neurosurgeons who had grown complacent, accustomed to diagnosing brain death and quietly reducing the level of care, were discomfited by family members requesting that the organs still functioning be donated before they failed, prodding them to do the needful to make transplantation happen. Nothing like this had ever been experienced anywhere else in the world!

Raza was excited by what he had found out and pieced together from the internet. There was hope, and not just a glimmer, a beacon!

The mood was not the same with Kunju. He wanted no part of this entire scheme. How could you possibly have somebody else's organ in your body, he wondered. Would he look different? What if he felt totally different? Changed in some fundamental way? After all, didn't they say the liver was the most important organ in the body, and controlled things like the emotions? What would Ayesha think of such a scheme?

Ayesha was quick to reassure him that he need not worry about any change in their relationship and feelings for each other. She had heard that after a transplant some people reported minor changes in their tastes and food preferences, but there was no major emotional alteration. A friend in Bangalore had told her about someone they knew who had undergone a heart transplant in the UK, and how he had not changed at all, other than becoming more energetic and this had actually made his family life a lot better. In fact she had been thinking about finding out where that heart transplant had been done and then taking Kunju to the same center. What her brother in New York had said about rules that prevented transplants for foreigners had put her plans on hold.

Meanwhile she was resigned to getting ready for their consultation in the Transplant Center to which they had been referred. She did not have the same enthusiasm that her children Raza and Shehnaz had with all their computer based researches, but she was determined to remain optimistic.

Two things were immediately noticeable to the Aliyar Kunju family as they arrived at the Transplant center. First, there were several individuals walking around with face masks, and second, finding a parking spot was going to be a big problem. Both Raza and Shehnaz enjoyed driving, and when they were home Ayesha would give Mustafa leave. After dropping his father, mother and sister off at the front entrance, Raza spent the better part of half an hour trying to find a parking place before finally giving up and handing over the keys to the Valet service – something he did not like to do normally. Mustafa's leave was cancelled to his barely concealed delight.

The first consultation was with the Transplant Coordinator who gave them a quick run down about the procedures planned. It would be a busy 2 days, and they could choose to get admitted, or to go and come from home – which was a reasonable option as they did not live far away.

The Coordinator, a young man who spoke Malayalam with a non-Malayalee accent had a stack of forms filled out for Kunju to sign, starting with the consent to undergo evaluation for transplantation. He said they would be meeting several people who were part of the "Transplant Team". Each person had a specific role to play, and at the end of the evaluation there would be a meeting of all members to decide whether he could be transplanted or if something needed to be fixed before transplant.

After the Transplant Coordinator, their first stop was the lab where they drew so much blood Ayesha found it hard to control herself from screaming at them to stop.

They soon realized that Kunju was going to get the most complete check-up that he had ever had in his life. All his organ systems would be evaluated by specialists, starting with his head. There would be liberal use of the fancy state of the art equipment of which there seemed to be no short supply.

The Ear Nose Throat (ENT) doctor was a young lady who, when Kunju mentioned he occasionally had a cough since he stopped smoking about 5 years earlier, promptly put a flexible fiberoptic scope into his nose and down the back of his throat to look into his vocal chords and larynx. The procedure was done in the out-patient clinic after spraying his nose with a local anesthetic to make it numb. The scope was much thinner than the one used to look into his stomach, but Kunju had no recollection of that, and this experience brought involuntary tears to his eyes as he tried to control gagging and vomiting. If there was a blood vessel waiting to burst in his head, it would most certainly have obliged right there in ENT.

From ENT, he was taken to Pulmonary lab where he had his pulmonary functions checked by breathing into a machine that recorded his various lung volumes. The respiratory therapist they met there was a young Muslim lady who wore a head scarf over her surgical scrubs. She was quick to make friends with Ayesha and Shehnaz, and told them privately that Kunju's lung functions looked OK, but he would need to start doing breathing exercises regularly.

Next it was the cardiology lab, where they made Kunju walk on a treadmill while recording his EKG. He found that his exercise tolerance could be measured and quantified. He was barely within the acceptable range, and was visibly exhausted by the end of the testing. For a former athlete it was terribly embarrassing. How had he allowed himself to slip like this, he wondered.

In the afternoon, after lunch in the cafeteria at the Transplant Center, the family headed over to the out-patient clinics to see the Hepatologist.

The Hepatologist, a former Professor, was in his 60s. He wore a tie, and a long somewhat crumpled white lab coat with a front pocket displaying the tops of a selection of pens. Raza spotted a Waterman in the collection – probably reserved for signing important documents, he thought. Other pockets contained various implements of his trade – a heavy stethoscope, a tuning fork, a pocket torch, a knee hammer that looked like a tomahawk, and even a little writing pad. He sat behind a desk in his consulting room with one desk top and one laptop computer, and as though to complete the theme of excessive preparedness, he had two pairs of glasses which he kept switching – one to read, and another to look at the computer screen. While talking to people he would look over the rim of whichever pair he was wearing at that moment.

Raza and Shehnaz had been giving various people nicknames so it would be easy to remember them afterwards. They named the Hepatologist "Dr. E" for Einstein, as he reminded them of the famous physicist, with his white moustache, bushy eyebrows, and mane of untidy white hair that spilled over his collar, and also because he introduced himself as a 'physician' confusing them initially because they thought they heard him say 'physicist'.

They would soon get used to the fact that there was a sharp distinction in roles between physicians and surgeons. Gone were the days, it seemed, when one doctor was able to do everything.

The time Dr. E spent with Kunju was the most that any doctor had ever spent on him in his life. The history he took seemed to probe into every aspect of his life including his eating habits, diet preferences, his daily activities, travel, family history, every single illness he had ever had, the drugs he took. Kunju felt he had never told anyone more about himself. Only when the entire 'history' was taken and recorded did the physical examination start. Starting at the top of his head and working down and all around, every part of his body was examined and every orifice it seemed, was probed. By the end of it Kunju felt Dr. E knew him better than he knew himself.

The family, who were waiting outside were called into the consulting room at the end of the examination, for a 'family conference'.

Yes, Dr. E said, their father needed a liver transplant. There was no question about this in his mind, but if they had questions, this was the time to ask.

Ayesha was suddenly reticent, unaccustomed to speaking openly with a stranger. Raza and Shehnaz had no such inhibitions, and the doctor seemed to encourage them. Later she tried to scold them saying they had not been respectful to the Professor and had talked too much, but to Kunju's delight, they scolded her right back.

"He's our Dad" they said, "if we don't get all the information we need to make sure he is safe, then who will?"

Kunju's sudden illness had brought the family together, and they were working and thinking like a team. It made him feel strong at a time when he should have been feeling weak.

They had learned a lot, and the children had made notes for later clarification, which they did, as father and mother rolled their eyes, ….. on the internet.

The blood tests, Dr. E told them, had ruled out viruses as the cause of Kunju's cirrhosis. Sometimes, a virus picked up earlier in life would lie dormant in the liver, and damage it slowly. The two main culprits were Hepatitis virus B called HBV for short, and Hepatitis virus C, or HCV. It was important for family members to know this, as viruses could affect multiple members in the same family, and detecting the traces of a hepatitis virus in one would be reason to look for it in all the others. Fortunately, this would not be necessary for the Aliyar Kunju family.

There were other diseases that could run in families, like Wilson's disease and hemochromatosis. Fortunately these were also ruled out in Kunju's case.

They had looked for 'autoimmune diseases'. These were conditions in which the immune system acted against the liver and damaged it. This group of conditions could affect other organ systems as well. It was important to find this out, as this made the subsequent management different, even after a transplant. Kunju had tested negative for these as well.

So why had he developed cirrhosis?

Dr. E said that he thought the most likely explanation was a diagnosis of exclusion, called NASH, short for 'non alcoholic steato-hepatitis'. The liver could get invaded by fat. This made the liver swell and become yellow in color. This was a common response to many toxic substances, and the most common toxic substance that caused this was, of course, alcohol.

In Kunju's case, alcohol was not involved, hence the term 'non alcoholic steatohepatitis'.

'Steato' meant 'fat', and hepatitis mean 'inflammation of the liver'. For as yet unknown reasons, in some people, liver fat was associated with inflammation, and this could progress exactly like the damage associated with alcohol, or viruses, or autoimmune disease.

And what exactly is cirrhosis?

Dr. E explained cirrhosis as scarring. Normal liver cells had been replaced by scar tissue. Had they seen anyone with excessive scar tissue? Dr. E reached into a drawer and brought out a picture of a girl with thick scars on her neck causing her neck to contract so severely that her chin was fused with her chest, making it impossible for her to look up, and extremely difficult for her to eat and breathe. Sometimes scar tissue seemed to acquire a life of its own, and would not stop growing, even invading the normal structures away from where it originally arose. Dr. E then showed them a picture of a cirrhotic liver. There was a picture of a normal liver also, for comparison. The cirrhotic liver looked ugly, yellowish brown, shrunken, distorted, and covered with nodules of different sizes that looked like excrescences. It was difficult not to shudder with disgust, just looking at the picture.

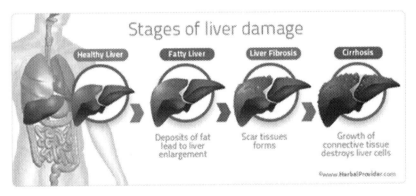

Stages of liver damage caused by fat accumulation in the liver

Figure 2: Stages of liver damage caused by fat accumulation in the liver. Fatty liver can be diagnosed on ultrasound scan. As it progresses, the blood vessels within the liver are increasingly difficult to visualize. The liver function tests become abnormal and this is sometimes a reason to do a liver biopsy. The stages of fibrosis and cirrhosis can be diagnosed by a biopsy. (Picture taken from www.HerbalProvider.com, used with permission)

As a result of the shrinking and scarring, blood could not easily transit through the liver on its way back to the heart, located just above the liver, and separated from it by the diaphragm. This caused blood to back up in the intestines, and that could of course, result in torrential haemorrhage.

That's what had happened to Kunju.

Another complication was cancer. With time, cancer could develop within the nodules. It was necessary for all patients with cirrhosis to undergo regular check-ups to see if cancer had developed within the cirrhotic liver. In fact some people did not know they had cirrhosis until the cancer developed, by which time it was too late. It was therefore necessary to do blood tests and scans on all patients with cirrhosis twice a year at least for the rest of their lives, or until they got a liver transplant.

When cancer developed, a whole new set of problems had to be dealt with. Dr. E said that he would not go into all that at this time since it was not applicable to Kunju.

This was a lot of information to take in at one time. The whole family sat dumb and dismal, staring at Dr. E.

Yes, he said, he knew it was all too much for any normal person to have to deal with. Unfortunately some people went into 'denial' which is the natural response to sudden bad news. They would ignore the diagnosis, and try and get back to their normal life. Family members would try to help and encourage, saying things like, "Oh you look fine!", "Don't worry!" or much more dangerously "try some other system of medicine. These allopathic solutions are too drastic...."

"But why do you say that another system like Ayurveda is dangerous, doctor?" asked Ayesha, "We have all heard that they have good medicines for curing liver disease!"

Shehnaz and Raza were surprised to see their mother had recovered her voice and her wits before them. They knew this question had been on her mind ever since the initial diagnosis was made, and friends and neighbors had of course blitzed her with exactly the kind of advice Dr. E had just warned them about. They hoped he would not find the question irritating.

Nothing seemed to shake Dr. E's composure. He described the trials that had been done with Ayurvedic medicines in hepatitis and particularly in viral hepatitis for which these medicine were quite popular. There was some evidence that they worked to alter the course of the disease with symptomatic improvement, but no strong evidence that they could alter the final outcome. Hepatitis had consequently remained endemic in India just like in other countries including China and Korea, all of which had strong traditions in native herbal medicines.

Whatever various systems of medicines might claim, the fact is you had to ask questions as to the diagnosis or the exact condition that was being treated. There was a big difference between "hepatitis" which is what Ayurvedic medicines were commonly used for, and cirrhosis. Hepatitis is an acute condition that can and should recover to normal if complications did not occur, if the causative disease agent did not persist.

The cirrhosis Kunju suffered from was an illness that had never had an acute phase, but had slowly and silently destroyed his liver. Now there was scar tissue all over the liver, and no medicine invented by or known to man anywhere could remove scar tissue and replace it with the original normal, supple, healthy tissue.

"Think about people you have seen with thick scars. Sometimes these follow severe injury like deep burns scars, but sometimes these can follow trivial injuries. No medicine has been invented that can effectively treat those persons, and make scar tissue go away. The only hope is surgery, and in fact there is a separate specialty called Plastic Surgery developed to deal with these kinds of disfiguring scars"

Shehnaz remembered a classmate whose ears had developed keloids after being pierced for ear rings. Yes, it was true, they had tried all sorts of medicines and injections but the thick unsightly scars remained. She had taken to wearing a Hijab in public.

Shehnaz knew her attention was wandering, the way it often did in a classroom. She forced herself to pay attention to the discussion, conscious that Dr. E was actually trying to educate all of them, and not only her Dad. A sudden thought struck her.

"And you are saying that all this liver destruction was caused only by fat?" asked Shehnaz incredulously.

Dr. E took his own time to answer this question. He seemed to sink into a reverie, and got a distant look in his eyes.

When he finally started talking, it was almost as if he were talking to himself.

"You know, I get many patients with liver disease, and I have been in this business a long time. In the past we worried a lot about hepatitis B. Then a vaccine came along, and promised to completely eradicate HBV in due course of time, the way small pox and polio are eradicated in India now. Apart from people who could be vaccinated, there were those unfortunates who had already got the disease as babies or young adults. For them, antiviral medicines have now been developed and we can eradicate the B virus from that individual. Hepatitis C is still a problem, though, with no vaccine, and no reliable drugs to treat infected persons, but even this is going to change as we are on the verge of breakthrough. Alcohol is a straightforward problem. If they stop drinking they get well, or we can transplant them, if they don't, nobody can help them. With fatty liver, the problem is much more complex, and there are many things about it we don't understand yet."

In fact it was hard to call it a disease. It was a disease only if one could call a nearly ubiquitous finding a disease.

"When they developed ultrasound scanning in the 1980s," reminisced Dr. E, "we began to diagnose fatty liver. Lately we are seeing it in epidemic proportions".

And in fact, by the '80s, Indians *were* getting fat. Visibly fat.

By the 1980s, food shortages in India had more or less disappeared. The chronic starvation of the colonial era had been replaced by the Green Revolution, genetically engineered high yielding strains of grain powered by fertilizer and pesticide. Soon the White revolution of industrialized milk production followed. Cows yielding less than 40 liters of high fat milk a day were left with no self- respect.

Unannounced and undetected, in a land where beef consumption was banned by law, a chicken-and-egg revolution took place. Chicken meat became widely available as chicken production became industrialized. Hens that had never ever stood up in their cages, or even remotely considered walking outside them had the muscular thighs and breasts of avian champions, only much more succulent and 'juicy'.

Somebody must be playing 'fowl' said Dr. E, with a twinkle in his eye.

Shehnaz caught the pun, and giggled.

Nobody, continued Dr. E, encouraged by Shehnaz's quick response to his humor, was asking any questions as they happily chewed on chunky chicken every day. Asking too many questions could be construed as 'hen-pecking', he added, lugubriously!

This time they all laughed.

If some people were not getting enough to eat, it was because they could not afford the prices, not because there was no food. Photographs of malnourished children and villages full of starving people, only skin and bones, were now associated more with the African continent than Asia.

Various reports started coming in from around the world where Indians had emigrated, suggesting that people of the Indian subcontinent were more prone than other races to the ill effects of excessive food. Publications from UK, where there were large communities of Indians, many of whom were vegetarians and therefore considered less prone to the ill effects of the western diet, described people from the Indian subcontinent being much more prone than other communities to early onset heart disease. Nutrition experts blamed the consumption of *ghee* – clarified butter – that nobody else in the world ever ate, but was a favourite among Indians, both vegetarians and non-vegetarians.

In India, diabetes starting in middle age was no longer a disease of the affluent. In fact it became an epidemic. Entire surgical wards, usually general wards, were devoted to managing the complications of diabetes as toe, foot, and leg amputations became common. The heart disease associated with fat people started showing up in Indians in their 40s and early 50s, just as had been already reported in Indians overseas.

While initial attention was focussed on the ill effects of fat on the heart, the effect of fat in the liver was completely ignored.

The fact is that most people with fatty liver disease have no symptoms whatsoever. Most thought they were in good health. And in a culture where being fat was associated with health and prosperity, nobody was prepared to believe that obesity was not a good thing.

Excessive body fat had a whole host of problems: from diabetes, to heart disease to hormonal disturbances. There was evidence, however that all fat is not equally bad. The fat that Sumo wrestlers accumulate seems to be mostly under the skin, and in this location it did not seem to make them sick. But when fat accumulated around the middle, inside the abdomen, that was when it seemed to create the most disease. In these individuals, many of whom had a waist bigger in circumference than their hips, fatty liver could make the transition from being a mere curiosity seen incidentally on an ultrasound scan done for some other reason, to fatty liver *disease*.

Fatty liver *disease* had excessive fat in the liver cells, but unlike mere fatty liver, the blood tests called liver function tests were abnormal, and biopsy showed inflammation of the liver. This constituted the disease called 'non alcoholic steatohepatitis' or NASH.

"But my husband is not fat, doctor!" Ayesha protested indignantly, "just look at him! Who will say he is fat?"

"You are right, madam," Dr. E said mildly, diffusing her indignation, "he does not *look* fat. Partly this is because in his younger days he used to be an athlete. But his BMI is over 30 which puts him in the range of obesity, and his waist-hip ratio is over 1 which means a significant part of his excess weight is located in his abdomen. These numbers, these measurements, are as important or significant as measurements of the pulse or blood pressure. Nobody *looks* like they have high blood pressure. You can only find out if you actually measure it."

In fact, he went on to explain, studies had shown that the simplest measure of risk was just to check the circumference of the belly at the waist, where "waist" was defined as the narrowest point on the belly. A waist circumference of more than 40 inches in males and more than 36 inches in females was sufficient to diagnose "central obesity" and was associated with the risks common to obese persons, including diabetes and heart disease and of course fatty liver and fatty liver disease. In fact in Indians there were those who believed the cut off for males is only 35 inches.

At the end of the busy day, tired and happy to be back home, Ayesha prepared to retire after giving her family dinner. Her ears were still ringing with Dr. E's words. She had decided she did not like him. In fact she had irritatedly told Shehnaz during their dinner conversation to stop calling him Einstein.

But his words had affected her, she could not deny that. It used to be her custom to insist everyone eat well, heaping their plates for their first helping, and insisting they have a second helping or even a third. This night however, she had made no protestation when someone said Enough. In fact she found herself watching carefully to see they did not eat too much. She was going to make sure the whole family lost some weight. Especially the children. If they had inherited some tendency to liver disease from their father, it was important to avoid anything that might adversely affect their livers.

As she changed into her nightie, she rummaged in the bottom of the drawer where she kept her sewing materials and found a measuring tape. Glancing around quickly to see nobody was watching she wrapped the tape measure around her middle. She had not done this in years, regarding herself too mature now for the girlish fixation of measuring 'vital statistics'. When she looked at the measurement of her waist she almost gasped with the shock. Her waist now was 3 inches more than her *hips* had measured when she was eighteen!

The next day their first appointment was with the Nutrition specialist. Having arrived early the Aliyar Kunju family waited alone in the department, studying the names of the Nutritionists. All were female. While they waited for the Senior Nutritionist, the younger ones in the department trooped in one by one. They were all slim and pretty, Ayesha noted, thinking to herself that they seemed to know what to eat. She was not the only one who had noticed.

"This seems to be the best looking department in this hospital, don't you think, son?" Kunju said to Raza.

Raza immediately recognized the deeper meaning of what his father had said. It was macho, an effort at self-confidence. "That's the spirit, Dad!" he laughed.

Shehnaz and Ayesha who had no such sensibilities, rolled their eyes in disgust at their menfolk.

They were somewhat reassured to see that the Senior Nutritionist with the expansive name of Bhagyalaxmi, had not escaped the middle age spread, and also wore glasses.

This time the questions were directed at the most personal aspects of their home and family – their eating habits. Kunju had to confess he not only did not stick to the restrictions of a diabetic diet, he really had no idea what it was. Ayesha also realized she had been lax, and had even been facilitating his non-compliance.

Bhagyalaxmi had already studied Kunju's record with the recent notes made by Dr. E. She explained that since the cause of cirrhosis was fatty liver disease, they would have to learn to watch Kunju's diet lifelong, and learn to count the calories consumed and make sure he stayed within the daily allowed limit.

"Do you have a weighing scale at home?" asked Bhagylaxmi

They had to admit they did not.

"Yeah, I also grew up thinking the only time to check one's weight was at the Railway station," she said.

Ayesha laughed. Shehnaz and Raza wondered what the heck they were talking about.

Ayesha had to explain how when she was a kid she would pester her father every time they were in a Railway station to give her fifty paise to check her weight on the fancy weighing machines they used to have on railway platform. Lights would flash, a red and white disc would whirl, and after a lot of mysterious clicks and clacks a card would come out with the printed weight (barely discernible) on one side and a fortune (barely understandable) on the other. Her mother of course would refuse to weigh herself at the railway platform, and once when Ayesha asked why, her father said that mother thought it was against their religion! It was a long time before she realized he was having a joke at mother's expense.

They would have to get into the habit of weighing Kunju every day before transplant, and also every week afterwards. In time this could be changed to monthly weight checks, but it was most important to keep track on a regular basis.

Bhagyalaxmi explained the concept of BMI, and her explanation seemed to be easier to understand than what Dr. E had said the day before. She turned the screen of her desktop computer to face the family and started clicking on the keyboard to do a Google search for "BMI calculator". This was the easiest way to calculate one's BMI, and it would be a good idea if everyone knew their BMI. It was probably as important as checking one's BP, she said.

In the room, against one wall, was a scale to measure height. She asked Kunju to stand up and checked his height.

"Your height is 175 cm," she announced.

"What is that in feet?" he asked. Like many people he was more accustomed to thinking in feet than in centimeters when it came to height.

Reading off the scale, Bhagyalaxmi said, "That is 5 feet 9 inches."

Kunju was surprised. "I used to be 5 feet and ten inches," he said, "are you sure your scale is right?"

"When was the last time you measured your height?" she asked

Kunju could not remember when. Perhaps 20 years earlier, he thought to himself.

People could lose height with age, Bhagyalaxmi explained. This was because the discs between vertebrae shrank. There was also some loss of muscle tone around the trunk. Whatever the reason, it made it likely at the same weight to go from being merely "overweight" to "obese" based on BMI.

She gave Kunju a "target weight" that he should try to achieve, and should always keep in mind as his "ideal body weight" based on his height.

Recurrence of the original disease following transplant was always a big concern. In the context of liver cirrhosis and liver transplant, some diseases like hepatitis C would always recur in the new liver, and there was no good way to predict what the course would be. But diseases like alcoholic liver disease and fatty liver disease were possible to control, and it was important that this control is established before transplant. It would be best if Kunju started trying to lose weight before transplant so that he would have the diet habits in place to prevent weight gain after transplant and recurrence of fatty liver disease in his new liver.

Unfortunately losing weight was the most difficult thing anybody could do. Even people in good health found it difficult to lose weight, so it was not surprising that people trying to fight a disease simultaneously should find this task nearly impossible.

The risk of complications after surgery was known to be higher in obese individuals with a BMI over 30. Wound infections, and lung infections were the main problem, and if these were survived, then heart disease and joint problems could start afterwards.

"Have you heard about surgery for weight loss?" she asked.

Ayesha's attention had begun to wander, but suddenly she was alert. Weight and weight loss were boring subjects, but recently there had been more and more talk about getting operations done to fix the problem quickly. She had always wondered about this and had wanted to consult an expert. The problem she had was to find out about weight loss surgery without being considered a candidate for the procedure!

Opening a book from her shelf that looked like an atlas of surgery with very beautiful anatomy drawings, Bhagyalaxmi explained some of the surgical options. To Ayesha and Kunju all the options appeared fascinating, but from a personal point of view uniformly unattractive, even scary.

The Nutritionist seemed to agree. It was not safe to have any operation now as his liver was so sick, but these options may be necessary after transplant unless Kunju could control his weight with diet and exercise alone.

In fact the whole issue of timing surgical weight loss procedures in someone who needed a transplant was as yet an unknown area, and the subject of research. It was not clear whether such operations were best carried out before or after a transplant. In the context of kidney transplant, most people who were 'morbidly obese' were now advised to get the operation done while on dialysis and lose the extra weight before transplant. This course was too risky for people with cirrhosis of the liver who were waiting for a liver transplant. Some centers with a lot of experience both in bariatric surgery and liver transplant had proposed to do the weight loss operation at the same time as a transplant. At this time it was not known if this is safe or not.

"What about slimming medicines?" asked Shehnaz. She was one person in the family who had been rapt in her interest throughout the session. The whole subject of Nutrition, she thought, was extremely interesting.

"Highly inadvisable," came the short reply. Bhagyalaxmi went on to explain how drugs that caused weight loss had been implicated in liver disease and even liver failure and several reports had been filed of perfectly normal people taking these medications and ending up needing a liver transplant.

"These days there are many medicines available on the market making great claims. Some claim to be herbal and natural and hundred percent safe, but ultimately these are all unverified claims. Everything you eat goes to the liver, and it bears the brunt."

There it was again. The same warning they had heard the previous day from Dr. E about Ayurvedic herbal medicines affecting the liver adversely. This was scary, thought Shehnaz, resolving to carefully study every medicine and herb before accepting the claims being made about them. There was no easy way out when it came to preventing or treating fat and weight gain.

For his part, none of the surgical weight loss procedures described were attractive, Kunju decided. He said he would lose weight on his own.

Bhagyalaxmi was ready to send him on to Physiotherapy. She gave Ayesha her business card.

"Call me with any questions" she said, pleasantly addressing the whole family. She would be following up weekly by phone.

She knew they would need all the help they could get.

The Physiotherapy Department was in a section of the building that least resembled a hospital. The Chief of the department was an athletic young man who looked like a walking advertisement for his specialty. He introduced himself as Nair, with a firm handshake. Kunju thought he must have some military background as the two men sized each other up.

After taking a brief history during which he seemed impressed with Kunju's earlier athletic credentials, he summoned one of his assistants, who put him through a series of strength assessment exercises, and gave him a pictorial card with the outlines of the exercises Kunju could get started on.

Although the interaction seemed to be over, Kunju and Raza seemed interested in lingering, to look at the equipment in the gymnasium section of the department, and also to see the other patients who were there being put through their paces.

"Hello, I am Krishnan," said a pleasant voice behind them, "are you checking out the gym?"

Father and son turned around to see their visitor, and introductions were made.

Krishnan, who liked to be called Krish, was a middle-aged man with a puffy look, and prominent bags under eyes which were a startling blue-grey color. His skin was unnaturally dark in exposed area, and unnaturally light colored in the areas normally covered by his clothes. He was slightly breathless having just finished a session on the treadmill under the watchful eye of one of the assistants.

"I am a transplant patient. I saw you at the check-in counter yesterday while I was paying some bills, and couldn't help overhearing the clerk asking you questions. Sorry."

Kunju felt a slight embarrassment at the fact that a complete stranger could have found out this intimate medical fact about him.

"I know what you are thinking," continued Krish, "there is very little respect for privacy and confidentiality in Indian hospitals. But then, it may be my own inquisitiveness, I must confess. I am always on the lookout for people who are in the same boat as I am." He laughed.

Kunju and Raza were immediately captivated by the outgoing personality before them.

"Are you also a liver patient?" asked Kunju.

"Oh, no, no! No such luck!" laughed their new friend, "I am lower in the hierarchy. A mere kidney patient. Much lower on the totem pole, I am afraid."

"Why do you say that?" asked Raza.

"Oh it's just a joke. I am not being serious," continued Krish, "I just like to read PG Wodehouse to keep my spirits up. You know – laughing is good for health and all that. Not that it stopped me from getting kidney failure, but who knows, it's what has probably kept my heart going! Wodehouse has this story about people in a hospital competing to see who has the most serious disease. The sorriest patient is someone who is going through treatments that he cannot brag about!"

Raza had never heard of PG Wodehouse. He told himself he would have to remember the name and look it up on Google later. If a guy in a hospital could have a laugh at his misfortune remembering what this writer wrote, he must be something to check out.

Krish certainly had faced his share of misfortune and more. He was not at all shy to share his story, and they heard all about it over lunch that, after Ayesha and Shehnaz had also been introduced, they decided to have together at the hospital cafeteria.

Krish was waiting for his second kidney transplant. His first kidney had lasted 6 years, he said.

"What happened?" Shehnaz wanted to know.

Krish smiled at the innocence with which the loaded question was asked.

"You really want to know? It's a long story. It might put you off your lunch!"

"That's OK. I watch all the medical serials on TV. Grey's Anatomy, House, Scrubs, everything! I'm not scared of watching an operation. In fact I am hoping they will let me see Dad's operation!"

"Ha ha! They're not likely to let you do that, old girl," chortled Krish, almost choking on his food, "confidentiality rules and all that!"

Krish had first discovered he had something wrong with his kidneys during a routine medical check up. That must have been better than the way he found out about his liver, Kunju thought to himself. How boring, thought Shehnaz waiting for the excitement to start.

They first discovered he had high blood pressure, and in the course of investigating it, they found that his kidneys were not normal. He had protein spilling in his urine, his urea and creatinine were high on blood testing, and an ultrasound scan showed his kidneys were shrunken.

"Once they are shrunken and scarred, there's not much you can do about them," said Krish, who seemed to have a thorough knowledge about his condition.

Ayesha remembered what Dr. E had said about scar tissue in Kunju's liver.

"Didn't you want to try some Ayurvedic treatment?" she asked, unwilling still to give up that hope.

"Oh yes, I did!" said Krish, suddenly not his usual cheerful self. "It made me so sick, I almost died! First they gave me a lot of dietary restrictions. Which did work of course in improving my urea and creatinine, so I felt very encouraged. But there has to be something wrong about taking herbs and potions and then coming back to modern medicine and getting blood tests to see if they work! I started losing weight and was always tired. When I finally accepted that nothing other than a new kidney was going to help me, I gave up the herbs and powders. They can cause the blood levels of Allopathic medicines to change and mess up everything. In fact it is well known that epileptic drugs stop working if you take herbal preparations, and someone whose epilepsy is well controlled can die of continuous convulsions after taking herbal preparations."

This was news to Ayesha. She suddenly realized there was a lot to be studied before accepting the claims of various drug manufacturers.

"But to get back to answering Shehnaz's question about what happened to my transplanted kidney, I have to say that the mistake I made was to get caught in the snare of a kidney broker."

Soon after Krish had been found to have shrunken kidneys on the scan, he had been referred to a transplant center. At the time there were very few, and he decided to go to Bangalore where many people were going for transplants at the time. The hospital was very posh, everyone was very welcoming, and rushed around to make him comfortable. In fact he was told that he could take a house on rent and have dialysis at home while waiting for his transplant. Everything would be set up at home, and a dialysis technician would be at his disposal and convenience. No hassles of waiting his turn in a crowded dialysis center.

Later he found out that the house where the dialysis machine was set up and available to him for rent was owned by the Nephrologist!

He was then introduced to the broker. The broker told him that he could get his transplant done before his next dialysis was due! The efficiency of the system was dazzling! The broker had a list of donors – upto twenty in each blood group – with all their tests complete, including CT scans and angiograms. The cost of the kidney was negotiable, the broker said, don't worry, they could always find a donor for the price he could pay, and even find a financial services company to help him with a loan as well.

For Krish who was paying around a thousand rupees for every dialysis at the time, with three dialysis sessions per week, this appeared to be a very attractive option. Most importantly, he would not have to ask a family member to donate a kidney for him. He had refused to allow his children to be considered as donors, and his wife was of a different blood type.

The negotiations with the broker began. For the healthiest donors with "favourable anatomy", which was an euphemism for someone whose kidney was surgically easy to remove and to transplant, the cost could be as high as ten lakhs. For lesser amounts, donors who had been turned down at some centers could be made available. The reason for such disqualification was usually difficult anatomy of the kidney. At least that was what Krish was made to understand. Nothing wrong with the donor otherwise, he was assured.

Krish paid the highest price demanded for the 'best quality' donor. The broker completed all the 'paperwork' which included getting official permission from a government committee that met twice a month at the Vidhan Soudha. Krish never got to see the donor, only the paperwork, and an assurance from the doctors that the donor looked good and the blood tests done to check compatibility were all fine.

Later he would find out that the donor got only Rs 25000. This was the 'price' fixed by the system of brokers and doctors in Bangalore, and was based, they said, on the compensation that the government used to pay for loss of a single limb to people injured in accidents while using the public transport system.

What was even worse, he got hepatitis in the course of his transplant.

Later they would say that he could have got exposed to hepatitis during dialysis in Kerala, or from the blood transfusions they had to give him during the transplant operation. But Krish was convinced that he got it from the donor. It was the easiest thing in the world to fudge blood tests, and the most untrustworthy person in the whole system was obviously the broker. He had realized that from the very beginning, but once caught in the tentacles of the 'system' he could not get out of it.

Later, Krish said, he realized that there was an essential paradox in someone being so poor that he had to sell his organs, and yet being fit enough to go through with it. Why would someone who was a hundred percent fit want to sell his kidneys for money? There were easier ways to make money after all!

"Rob a bank, for God's sake!" Krish hooted with laughter! "if you get away with it, you don't need to lose a kidney! And if you get caught, hey the taxpayers are there to pay for your welfare in jail! Ha ha!"

The Aliyar Kunju family sat transfixed by the story of their new found friend. This kind of stuff was better than any Grey's Anatomy serial, thought Shehnaz to herself.

When his blood tests started going haywire, and his liver functions were at their worst about 6 months after the transplant, hepatitis C was diagnosed. They then tried to treat it, and he got a rejection of his kidney transplant. His creatinine which had come down to less than 1 soon after his transplant, began going up and never again dropped below 3. He had to go back to being super careful of everything he ate, once again reducing protein intake, Ayurveda style, to the bare minimum compatible with life to somehow desperately prolong the life of the transplanted kidney. But the inevitable had happened, and he was back on dialysis, and waiting for his second kidney transplant.

"At the moment, they say my liver is withstanding the effects of the hepatitis virus, so I may never need a liver transplant down the road, but who knows!

I may end up like you, on the top of the hierarchy! Numero Uno. Number One," laughed Krish. "No such luck this time, though! I just have to get fit to fight a second round!"

Krish's reference to boxing immediately resonated with Kunju. Never had he seen someone who was so resilient and tough, he marvelled. If this bantamweight could survive all that he had been through, and still laugh about it, the difficulty he was facing was well within his ability to conquer.

The last appointment for the day was for Kunju to meet the Transplant surgeon. Shehnaz and Raza were excited to meet a real transplant surgeon, but Ayesha and Kunju were apprehensive, not looking forward to this consultation at all.

The Chief Surgeon, who everyone called either Chief, because he was the chief, or Prof, because he used to be, like Dr. E, a university Professor, was the opposite of the usual surgical stereotype – neither tall nor imposing. In fact they mistook him for some junior member of the hospital staff, as he was dressed in hospital scrubs, with a surgical cap covering his head, and a mask dangling around his neck when he first walked past them in the waiting area to enter his consulting room. He was slim, short and walked with a slightly pigeon toed gait and short bouncy steps, looking as though at any moment he was ready to break into a run. When he came out carrying the clipboard with Kunju's medical chart, he wore his lab coat over his scrubs, and they could read his name and designation printed above the top pocket. Unlike Dr. E he had no pens whatsoever in the pocket. Also unlike Dr. E, he was cheerful, seeming perpetually amused and trying hard to be serious. He greeted the whole family, shaking hands with Kunju and Raza, and bowing courteously to Ayesha and Shehnaz, wishing them cheerfully good afternoon before walking Kunju into his consulting room. There was a lively, contagious confidence about him. Something about him reminded Raza of a certain comic character.

"Doesn't he remind you of Asterix?", whispered Raza to Shehnaz.

"Yes, he does!" she whispered back, barely able to control her laughter. "But he's not as ugly as Asterix!"

They were referring to the Gaul superhero who used to pound Roman soldiers into a pulp after drinking magic potion.

Thereafter they would refer to him as Dr. A.

"What do you think of him, Mom?" asked Shehnaz.

"I don't know," she said cautiously, thinking to herself that with his boyish looks he must have difficulty staying out of trouble.

With Kunju in the consulting room the rest of the family waited outside on tenterhooks. After about ten minutes, a nurse emerged to invite them into the room. They crowded in, apprehensive but eager to know what was going on.

"Your Dad, as you already know, needs a liver transplant," Dr. A started slowly, his laughing eyes serious as he watched their faces carefully, "and I like to keep the family involved at every stage. We, meaning your Dad and the surgical team, will need all the help we can get from you to get him safely through the operation and the post operative period. I have his permission to include you all in discussions, and you can ask me anything you want to know."

When asked to ask questions, patients and their families are usually unable to think of any. Dr. A had encountered such awkward silences many times and he ploughed on with his explanation of the transplant procedure.

First of all, he said, Kunju appeared to be a good candidate for surgery based on all the investigations they had undergone. Once the financial clearance had been obtained by the Finance section, he would be placed on the waiting list with KNOS, the Kerala Network for Organ Sharing, for a liver transplant. As and when a donor became available, he would be called in for the transplant. This could happen any day or night, and they had to be prepared to come into hospital at short notice.

It was hard to predict how long this waiting process would take. Different organs are allocated by different rules. In the case of kidneys, the time spent on the waiting list is given a lot of importance. However in the case of liver and heart, 'medical necessity' was the most important factor.

In other words, in the case of a heart or liver transplant, the person on the top of the list was the one most sick and at risk of dying compared to the others in the same blood group in that hospital or in that region. For every organ there was a system of calculating points, on the basis of which the position on the waiting list would be decided.

In the case of liver transplantation, the way to determine a patient's position on the waiting list is by calculating the 'MELD score'.

Dr. A turned to the computer on his desk, and pulled up Google, then put in a search for "MELD calculator". Raza and Shehnaz were immediately interested. Looking at Kunju's lab results on his clipboard, Dr. A put in the necessary data into each box, and then hit the 'calculate' key.

A score of 14 or over was the general guideline accepted worldwide, Dr. A said, to move a patient from medical management to liver transplant. It was now accepted worldwide that above a score of 14 a person's best hope was a transplant.

Kunju's MELD score was 27

"That's a high score," said Dr. A, suddenly serious, "it will put him near the top of the list in his blood group."

Raza and Shehnaz looked happy. Kunju, not so much.

"That means our Dad may get a transplant quite soon!" said Shehnaz.

"Well, I would like to say Yes," said Dr. A, "but that would not be completely correct".

In countries where organ donation after death was well established, it is actually possible to figure out the average waiting time for someone with a MELD score that high, but as yet, in Kerala it was not possible to do so as the program was still being established.

The family looked crestfallen, their hopes dashed. This was going to be like waiting for a lottery!

"I have to tell you there is an alternative," said Dr. A, cautiously. "Mr. Aliyar Kunju and I have already discussed it."

The alternative was to have a live donor transplant, but only an immediate family member or close blood relative was permitted by law to be the donor. In some parts of India where cadaver organ donation was not developed, only people with a suitable live donor who matched the patient in blood group and size could be transplanted.

However, they were lucky to be in Kerala, as here the public was beginning to support donation after death, and since establishment of the Kerala Network of Organ Sharing, called KNOS or Mrithasanjeevani, the number of organ donations had shown a steady increase.

"I am ready to donate my liver," said Raza to Dr. A.

"That is good Raza, a brave and noble gesture," answered Dr. A, "but I have already gone over this with your Dad, and he has said he would like to go for a cadaver donor organ as his first choice. We can however do some basic work up on you and keep you ready as a stand by should the transplant be urgently required for any reason. But I want you all to think about it some more before we proceed."

"Tell me more about this, doctor," Raza insisted, "why are you not considering me as the first choice. Don't listen to my Dad. I want to be his donor."

"Me too," said Shehnaz.

"No Raza," Ayesha said, with a stern note in her voice. "And you Shehnaz, don't even think about it! I am the first one to be the donor for your father. You children have your life before you."

Dr. A listened to the family argument in silence. He seemed to be lost in thought.

"You know, a couple of years ago we would have immediately proceeded to work on finding out which one of you would be the best donor for your father. There was no other choice in most Asian countries."

First performed in Australia on a Japanese national, and later popularized in Japan, liver transplantation was revolutionized in the '80s and '90s using a segment of liver from a living donor. Using live donors for children had become established first, and had proved to be very successful all over the world, so that children rarely ever died these days on a waiting list.

Live donation for adults was slower to start. Because the amount of liver required to be removed from the donor was larger than needed for a child, this put the donor at greater risk. When a few donors died, the procedure became very controversial in the west, and some centers were closed by the government or denied permission to continue with adult-to-adult live donor liver (also called 'A2ALL') transplant.

In the west where transplant outcomes are closely monitored, cadaver organ donation continued to be the norm, and sufficient number of organs to meet the demand could be raised from organ donation after death. In Asia, however, the complex organization and public education required for such a program was not easy to establish. And A2ALL continued to find increasing application in Asia.

It soon became obvious that success depended on a lot of factors that were hitherto unknown. The first obstacle that was worked out was the size of the piece required to be taken from the donor. The critical metric was size matching the donor and recipient. If the donor was not physically of the same size or near about, it was not possible to get an adequate size of liver for an adult recipient. The weight of the piece of liver from the donor had to be about 1% of the weight of the recipient. In other words if a recipient was about 70 kg, then the size of liver required was 700gm. The minimum would be 0.8% or about 560 gm. Oriental Asians were small built generally, and more uniform in size than in the west, so finding a size matched donor was easier than in other countries and races.

The next factor influencing live donor liver transplantation was the quality of the donor's liver. Since only a part of the liver was being used it was imperative that it be normal.

"A big problem encountered in potential living liver donors is 'fatty liver'", said Dr. A. "It is too risky to both donor and recipient to take a segment of liver from someone with more than 15% fat. In India this has been a big problem, as we seem to have more fatty liver disease than is seen in countries like Japan and Korea."

There it was again. The new 'F word': Fatty liver. Ayesha was convinced if she heard it again she would scream.

In the past assessing the amount of fat in someone's liver was difficult and often erroneous. Now there were better ways of finding out the percentage of liver fat, and a test called MRI spectroscopy was currently considered the standard. Unfortunately, the kind of MRI scanner required for this was not available everywhere. Ultrasound scans, CT scans and sometimes liver biopsy were necessary.

The last important factor in the decision whether to go for a whole liver from someone who has died, or a partial liver from a living donor is the MELD score of the recipient. With living donors, the best results were if the recipient's MELD score was 18 or less. Of course if someone required an emergency transplant, this consideration would have to be relaxed.

"You mean even if my liver is big enough for Dad, you will not use it if his MELD score is high?" Raza had not yet given up his idea of being the donor for his Dad.

"There are some centers that would," answered Dr. A. "What I would advise is that we put your father on a cadaver waiting list first, and complete your check up so you are ready, should the need arise. Meanwhile we can work to optimize your father's condition and see if his MELD score comes down, thus giving him more options."

Clearly, this was a complex decision, not to be rushed. They would have to think seriously about it, and were lucky that Kunju did not need liver transplant as an emergency.

"Any more questions?" asked Dr. A.

"Isn't it risky to get an organ from someone you do not know at all, doctor?" asked Shehnaz. "We just met someone who got hepatitis from his donor during a kidney transplant. That is so frightening."

Dr. A nodded immediately, "Good question," but took his time to reply.

Yes, it was always possible to get disease from an organ donor. No transplant program anywhere in the world could guarantee zero risk. However, the good news was that the screening tests to detect infectious diseases were getting more and more accurate. What had become apparent, though, was that the critical thing was to get a good medical history from family members of the person who had died. Unlike brokers and paid donors, these people had no reason to conceal anything. People who donate organs after death had come to hospital for treatment of a head injury or a primary condition of the brain, and a complete history and all the necessary investigations for common communicable viruses would have already been obtained at the time of admission, making it unlikely that anything was missed. Nevertheless at the time of donation everything was double checked, and tests not done were done and anything that was equivocal was checked again before proceeding to organ donation. So, although time was not unlimited, the screening for infections was actually better and more reliable than in the past, when unrelated and impoverished live donors being herded by mafia-style brokers was the norm.

Lastly, unlike paid kidney donors, donation after death requires a complete autopsy be performed, and this is another safety check for any sign of disease in the donor.

Shehnaz looked relieved.

"There will be more questions, as you learn more," said Dr. A. "That is only natural. Remember we are here to answer all your questions. I will ask Raza to see our Hepatologist to do the preliminary checks to see if he can be an organ donor. For now, however it is most important to complete all the formalities and get onto KNOS's waiting list. You never know when you will get a good donor offer, and we have to maximize the chances of that. Luck favors those who are prepared."

Raza's consultation with Dr. E., was brief. He was in and out in 5 minutes.

"What happened?" asked Aysha.

Raza looked glum.

"I am overweight," he said. "I've been told to lose 10 kg before Dr. E will agree to even do any tests on me."

Kunju and Aysha did not know what to think or say. They had mixed feelings. Most dominant was the fear that Raza might obviously be prone to the problems that had affected Kunju. But secretly they were relieved their son would not be undergoing surgery to donate part of his liver.

"That's OK, son", they said, "don't worry about it."

"What do you mean, 'don't worry'?" Raza snapped indignantly, "of course I need to worry. For starters I am going to lose weight. They've given me 3 months to lose 10 kilos. I am going to start running tomorrow. And Mom, no rice, and no chicken for me. Please!"

Mustafa was excited as he brought the car around to the hospital entrance. Pointing with his chin and eyes, as he opened the door for Kunju to get in, he directed everyone's gaze to the rear entrance of the parking lot.

"See that ambulance parked there?" he said, "they brought a kidney from a hospital in Kottayam! It is going to be transplanted here! I spoke with the driver. The same driver had gone out on rescue, and picked up the accident victim from the roadside. He was saying the head was badly injured, he had never seen so much blood in his life! He had to drive like hell to get to the hospital fast, but they couldn't save the poor chap. All organs were donated by the family in Kottayam this morning, and it seems the heart was rushed to Kochi with a police escort! You must check the news tomorrow. It will be in the papers!"

Ayesha was not sure she should be happy about the whole story the way Mustafa was. Silly man, getting all dramatic. This was somber news. Think of the family of the poor donor!

And yet, she could not deny that something good had come of the tragedy.

"One day Sir will also get his transplant", Mustafa enthused, referring to his beloved boss in respectful third-person, "I am sure of it!"

When they sat down for supper that night, they had to acknowledge that Mustafa, and his humble faith that everything was going to work out, had made their mood significantly better. No longer were they even subconsciously thinking about their predicament as 'bad luck'.

PART II

THE WAIT

With siren screaming, and overhead lights flashing, the ambulance sliced through traffic, rushing towards Kochi down the National Highway. Heavy trucks hogged the fast lane forcing the ambulance to careen into the slow lane and overtake dangerously from available space on the left side. An occasional car quickly moved over to the extreme left side of the road to let the ambulance pass. Most however refused to yield space or change lanes.

Chaotic traffic with everybody a law unto himself is the norm on Indian roads, and Kerala despite its distinction of nearly 100% literacy was no exception. People either did not know, or did not care about the principle, accepted universally, that emergency vehicles are to be given right of way on the road.

The ambulance driver cursing almost continuously, ploughed on.

Inside, strapped to a stretcher and fighting for his life, was an accident victim, found lying on the road, hit by an unknown vehicle which had fled the scene. Ironically, the patient would also be labeled "Unknown" at admission, because nobody knew who he was. The ambulance was part of a network provided for by the Rotary club, and positioned at strategic points along the highway – usually close to stretches of road that traffic police statistics had recognized as "Accident Prone".

Apart from the constant swerving, the ride was bumpy as potholes were unavoidable, and 'speed breakers' ubiquitous. Rumor had it that the arbitrariness with which speed breakers were constructed could be explained by the fact that people considered having a speed breaker outside their establishment a sign of importance and prestige.

The final bump was of course the speed breaker constructed at the entrance to the hospital itself!

Whether from the initial trauma of the road accident, or the bumpy ride that followed, the Casualty Medical Officer who saw "Unknown" immediately on arrival, knew his chances for survival were poor.

He was young, perhaps in his late twenties or early thirties, and appeared to have been in good physical condition prior to the accident. Shirt and trousers, tattered and bloody now, but of good quality, put him in the category of someone in the economic middle class. It was critical to determine this fact. Patients who looked like they would not be able to pay were best sent right on to the government hospital located another 20 minutes down the road.

Wheeled into the Casualty bay, the patient was in a coma, with no response to pain other than to groan and stiffen up with arms and legs extended and back arching in a powerful spasm, painful to behold. His eyes were puffed out with black discoloration around both orbits, and when the CMO pushed apart the swollen eyelids, the eyes were bloodshot with no area of normal white visible around the cornea. Shining a light into the pupils was again associated with a struggling effort as though to move away from the light and another groan. But the CMO had seen what he was looking for: the pupil was dilated and did not react to the bright light by constricting as they should. He repeated the test on the other side, and confirmed the same finding.

The blood pressure had meanwhile been taken by a nurse and was nearly normal. She quickly found a vein for a large bore iv line in the left forearm, and hooked up a bag of saline after drawing blood samples to send to the lab for routine tests, and to the blood bank to arrange blood for transfusion.

A code had been called the moment the accident victim reached the Emergency Room, and soon the resident Anesthetist on call was at the side of the CMO to help. They decided that the patient needed to be intubated and hooked to a ventilator before sending him to x-ray.

While the young doctors and nurses worked on the patient trying to do everything by the book, a darker side of Emergency Trauma Care in India was unfolding.

The nurse, enthusiastic to practice all that she learned in school, also had administrative responsibilities from which doctors in Casualty were spared. Accordingly, she informed the Nursing Supervisor on call about the arrival of "Unknown". A quick phone call was all that was necessary.

The Nursing Supe, a substantially older and substantially larger version of the young girl rushing around Casualty to try and save the patient's life, sighed audibly, and with a harassed look, folded the registers she was working on in her office. Reaching for the hook on which she had hung her impeccably starched white coat, she pulled it on over her colorful sari, carefully smoothing the opposing fabrics – silk sari and cotton coat – over the promontory of her substantial bosom before emerging from her office to wind her way downstairs to Casualty. She was in no hurry.

Outside the resuscitation area, she noted, there was no crowd of anxious relatives and excited onlookers, that normally accompany the arrival of a patient in the Casualty bay. No strenuous tussle was ongoing between hospital Security and "Bystanders", as patients' relatives are commonly referred to. Wrestling matches at the Casualty entrance are an integral part of the job of crowd control entrusted to the uniformed hospital security staff.

So routine, frequent, and expected were these loud encounters between Security and Bystanders, that most hospital buildings were designed to have their Emergency department at the rear of the hospital, so that chaotic scenes at the entrance were shielded from view of the more dignified, sedate patients who came in through the Main Entrance to get their more dignified and sedate conditions treated in orderly fashion by dignified, sedate and much more senior doctors than the young crew manning the Emergency area.

For Nursing Supe, the peace and quiet today was troubling.

Wandering through the deserted Casualty – everyone it seems had rushed off to help in the resuscitation area – she made her way to where the action was, with increasing apprehension. Her entrance had gone unnoticed, and she was content with that, as she needed to be invisible as far as possible to complete the task uppermost in her mind.

She was there to try and determine who "Unknown" was, and more importantly whether he and his family – whenever they showed up - were likely to afford the cost of all the medicine being poured into and onto him, the expensive scans, xrays, and ICU care that would most certainly follow. The judgment of Casualty medical officers was notoriously poor in this critical area of medical practice.

The tattered clothes of the patient, cut away in the course of resuscitating him, have to be retained in a sealed cover for subsequent production in court as exhibits, should the need arise. Nursing Supe had the responsibility to make sure the necessary medico-legal formalities were properly completed during the rush and bustle of Emergency care. Before sealing the bag, she would go through the pockets to try and find some lead – an ID badge, the address on a letter, a cleaner's bill – anything that might help identify the accident victim and perhaps enable his family to be contacted. They were needed at the bedside to help with care, and also, importantly, to pay for it.

Emergency Trauma Care was expensive. At the very minimum it worked out to a thousand rupees an hour, often four or five times that amount to start, and that was the kind of money the hospital was hemorrhaging at this time on this patient, with no hope of recovering the amount.

The 'milk of human kindness' – that Shakespearean prerequisite of mercy – had long since been wrung out of the generous bosom of Nursing Supe, by the practical realities of her job. In the frequent, almost daily, balancing act between bloody hemorrhage in a patient, and monetary hemorrhage of the institution that employed her, Nursing Supe knew on which side to throw her considerable weight.

This "Unknown" lying there in the resuscitation bay and sucking up hospital resources by the minute, might end up dead before any of his relatives could be found. Relatives showing up when the body was in the mortuary do not generally take kindly to paying a hospital bill of several thousands of rupees.

What would happen tomorrow if there was an even bigger pile up on the highway, and half a dozen trauma victims were brought in? Could the hospital be expected to extend free care to them as well?

And God forbid a government owned vehicle or a State Transport bus was responsible for the broken and crushed person lying bleeding before her! Union workers had made sure nobody could be held responsible for the accident. Then, could anyone be held responsible to pay the hospital bill? Never! Even in the unlikely event that a court of law would order such payment to be made.

She comforted herself in the knowledge that when nobody seemed to care about the epidemic of trauma in India which she had been seeing ever since she too was a young nurse, she could not be expected to do anything to fix the badly broken system. It was the duty of the government to fix the problem, she was fond of saying.

She was right.

Successive governments had come and gone, but the problem of managing the greatest epidemic in India had remained. The underlying reality in Indian electoral politics was the "anti-incumbency factor", a unique term coined in India to describe the tendency of frustrated voters to throw out the incumbent party in governance each time elections came around. So pervasive was this reality, and so fundamental to all negotiations, that everybody understood and accepted that the only real consideration of the party in power was to make their money and run. Hopefully they would make enough to cover the expenses of the next election and get voted back into power, although paying for votes was never a sure strategy for success any more.

When newly independent from colonial Great Britain, and flushed with socialistic idealism, the Constituent Assembly of India in 1948 had created one of the first pieces of social security legislation ever enacted in the world. It was called the Employee State Insurance (ESI) Act. Like all countries recovering from the devastation of World War II, and wondering how the Germans could have resurrected themselves to be such a powerful country so soon after the near total destruction of World War I, India also looked at the social security insurance systems introduced in Germany to pay for health, disability, trauma, and sickness. Having social security was recognized as an essential ingredient to the overall efficient performance of the work force.

Inherently comfortable with the realities of a rigid caste system, even while paying lip service to ideals of socialism and *egalite`*, the government had extended social stratification into the social security system of India. The ESI act applied only to Government employees and factory workers. Nobody else had really mattered during the colonial era. The so-called socialist system that replaced colonial rule was blind to the caste system that had developed within social security.

If you didn't work for the government, or some factory, you looked after yourself. You were expected to save enough money for your medical treatments, the accidents that may befall you, and for your retirement. Nobody else was responsible.

The problem nobody anticipated in 1948, was the growth of the automobile industry in India. Scooters, motorcycles, rickshaws, autorickshaws, pick up trucks – some with three wheels and some with four, massive lorries with twenty four wheels, buses with drivers in a mad hurry to overtake other buses in competition for passengers waiting ahead, and cars whose drivers (often retired from bus service, and retaining their competitiveness) did not want to be outdone, competed for space on narrow Indian roads designed for the width of bullock carts. Pedestrians, cyclists and cattle trying to make it on their own steam got no respect, and expected none, crossing roads where they felt like, not so much because they were in a hurry, but to save what they could of their limited stores of energy. Global warming coupled with smog raised the heat, sapping everyone's patience, an incendiary mix that resulted in an accident rate that grew exponentially every year. People were maimed and killed on a daily basis in a mind numbing upward statistical spiral.

By the '90s India's citizenry had tired of the socialist experiment of the previous fifty years. With the economy becoming increasingly unfettered, India went into economic overdrive. Cities grew in unplanned spontaneity, even as successive governments still stuck in a socialist mindset and fond of 'five year plans', diverted development funds to villages, large wads of which found their way back to private accounts in city banks.

Medical services emerged out of the shadow of government run hospitals stuck in the middle ages, as 'corporate hospitals' run for profit and organized on strict business principles took off. Most of these focused on diseases that required expensive and specialized services of an elective nature. Cancer, heart disease, laparoscopic surgery, Urology, Gastroenterology, and Plastic surgery services were developed. The essential feature common to all these specialty hospitals was that the conditions they diagnosed and treated, permitted treatments to be conducted in a leisurely manner, allowing patients enough time to raise the necessary funds.

Emergency services and particularly Trauma care were left behind. Malodorous government hospitals, mired in a time warp of bureaucratic bungling and administrative inefficiency, overflowed with desperately poor people laid out on rickety iron cots or hastily spread sheets on cement floors within, while anxious relatives camped outside on sidewalks and gardens outside. These were the designated providers of Trauma care expected to cope with the greatest epidemic the country had ever encountered.

Study after study showed that most civilian Trauma deaths and injuries were caused by accidents involving vehicles on the road, and most of these occurred in urban areas. However, accident victims had no rescue system in most cities and the kindness of passersby was required to take them to a hospital. Despite this, amazingly, the first contact with medical care almost always occurred in the first hour – the "golden hour" – such was the good neighborliness of common folk in India. But this was not necessarily matched by the medical establishment. Study after study showed that the time taken for definitive treatment to start in Trauma cases was much longer: 4 to 6 hours on average, and upto 12 hours at some megacities.

Frustration with the system was widespread, and directed against hospitals and the medical fraternity who were blamed for neglecting accident victims. In 1989 a landmark judgment of the Supreme Court made it compulsory for 'all government hospitals and medical institutions' to provide 'medical aid' to accident victims. Privately run hospitals responded by providing band-aid dressings on head injuries for patients who could not pay on the spot, and sent them on to 'higher centers' for 'higher level of care' with a note saying 'Neurosurgeon not available'.

(The honorable judges of the Supreme Court had neglected in their judgment, to order Neurosurgeons to be available).

In the absence of any system to pay for immediate and expensive care that involved taking scans inserting expensive iv cannulas, administering expensive oxygen and then, in most cases, anesthesia for emergency surgery, and post operative ICU care with ventilators and what-not, private hospital administrators quietly introduced avoidance tactics that had 'cut the losses' as the guiding principle in the provision of Trauma care.

Not a single city, with the possible exception of some areas of Mumbai - the commercial and movie capital of India, had an organized system of roadside rescue. Trauma centers designated by level of expertise available, did not exist in any city. There were no clear instructions to ambulances as to where they should go with a trauma victim. Bus stations, railway stations and airports proliferated with no plans for where they would take casualties in the event of a crash and sudden mass casualties.

Not that there was any shortage of money for this purpose.

In a twist of irony the only people in India who had an unlimited store of insurance money to take care of them were the victims of vehicular trauma.

The Motor Vehicles Act had made it compulsory for all vehicles to carry "third party insurance" while plying on a public road. A study in the 1980s in the megacity of Bangalore with a population of 7 million at the time, estimated that there were one and a half million two-wheelers on the road. At the time the third party insurance premium for two wheelers was Rs 100 per year, making over Rs 150 million available for trauma care from two wheelers alone.

Since then the population had multiplied to almost double, while insurance premiums for vehicles had more than quadrupled. It was a fair estimate that billions of rupees were now being collected by government owned and operated insurance companies from compulsory third party vehicle insurance meant to pay for accident victims.

Where was this money going?

In fits of misguided legislation, aimed perhaps at preventing insurance money due to accident victims being siphoned off by "vested interests", government had decided this money was to be made available through tribunals, called the Motor Vehicles Tribunals.

Accident victims had to be present personally or represented by an attorney at the Tribunal. Calculation of the amount of compensation depended on proving to the Tribunal that the victim had suffered a "permanent disability" on the basis of which some compensation would be negotiated. In the case of death the amount disbursed would take into account the loss of potential earning.

A network of lawyers 'specializing' in accident cases developed. Large trauma centers had lawyers openly parked outside in vans from which they provided desperate family members seemingly large sums of money as 'loans' to pay for treatment, in return for signing a legal document employing their services for representation before the Motor Vehicles Tribunal. The lawyers, in collaboration with insurance agents and the Tribunal 'settled' on compensations from which their fees were extracted before giving the victim the residue.

The sums of money thus awarded could be very large, and the larger the claim the longer the judicial process. There was no time limit for the process, and appeals could take years as thousands of lawsuits wound their way through an overburdened judicial system of lower courts, high courts and appellate courts. It was not unusual for an award to be finally made 6,

10 or 15 years after the accident occurred, with the insurance company that had insured the vehicles involved fighting bitterly all the way and finally parting reluctantly with their money.

By which time hospital expenses, if left unpaid at the time of the accident, were forgotten.

The system was designed not to care for, but to compensate victims of vehicular accidents.

Every privately owned hospital with available trauma care facilities knew this, and could do nothing about it. The only hope was to somehow quickly figure out on arrival which patient would be able to pay for the facilities, and hold onto them, while sending the less fortunate ones packing, after "first aid" of course, to the nearest government facility. Never mind the deleterious effects of the secondary transfer and the delay in starting definitive treatment. And never mind the fact that the Government Hospital to which the patient was transferred was too poorly equipped to provide decent trauma care.

This was what Nursing Supe was charged with doing, and had over the years become adept at. From her experienced assessment, in her learned opinion, this case was best transferred to a government hospital as soon as possible. She dug out her cell phone from the pocket of her white coat and dialed.

The phone rang in the office of the Senior General Manager, on the second floor of the Administrative section far removed from the scene of the most hectic activity, as Hospital Administrations tend to want to be.

The Sr.Manager was a youthful former Army major, retired after a short but hectic service in the Army Medical Corps. Maj. Dr.Deepak Nair, or

Major Deepak as he liked to be called, had recently been appointed to his post and charged with the task of improving operations ("Ops", he called it) all around.

"Good Morning Sister Cecily!" he boomed into the phone. Having insisted his phones be fitted with caller ID, he enjoyed the immediate imbalance caused to the person at the other end, who was startled to find that self-introduction had been miraculously rendered superfluous.

"Good morning Sir. I am Nursing Supervisor speaking," Nursing Supe continued, not immediately cognizant of the fact that she had been greeted by name even while she thought she was still anonymous. She taught telephone manners to her nurses, and took the lessons seriously herself: always identify yourself on the phone. It was of course understood that divulging your name was optional as you rose in rank.

"Yes, Sister" Maj. Deepak acknowledged, understanding from her tone that this was going to be a serious conversation "What can I do for you?"

"There is an Unknown brought to Casualty, Sir," Nursing Supe was not going to beat around the bush, "we have to send him immediately to the government hospital. I need your permission to use our hospital ambulance."

"Ambulance. Hospital ambulance," Maj. Deepak repeated, "to government hospital."

Maj. Deepak had a habit of repeating the last words, or sometimes the gist of entire sentences he had just heard. It gave him time to collect his thoughts.

"It is urgent, Sir," Nursing Supe was in no mood to allow him to collect thoughts or anything else. Although he was higher than her in the hospital hierarchy, she was older and senior, and felt she was better than him at administration. He was in need of instruction. Her instruction.

"Urgent?" Maj. Deepak said, thinking to himself he probably definitely had to delay this request.

"Yes urgent," said Nursing Supe, a great repetition artist in her own right.

"Urgent. But can I ask, what is wrong with the patient, Sister?" Maj. Deepak asked pushing the exchange forward.

"I told you, Sir. He is an Unknown!" Nursing Supe was getting a little shrill.

"Unknown. Unknown? Yes. You did say he is Unknown," acknowledged Maj. Deepak. "But what is wrong with him."

"Head injury, Sir. RTA!" short for 'road traffic accident'.

"RTA. Yes. But why not we treat him here, Sister? Our Neurosurgeon is not on leave. I can call him immediately" Maj. Deepak had, since he took over Administration at the hospital made significant strides in reducing sudden leave-taking, and had introduced an electronic check in system which not only marked attendance but let him know who were the chronic latecomers.

"But he is an Unknown, Sir", Nursing Supe's pitch was rising, "and they are wanting to shift him for CT scan!"

"CT scan. Yes. CT scan." Maj. Deepak repeated, "Yes, Sister, you have my permission to get the scan done."

Nursing Supe had not asked for his permission, and it was on the tip of her tongue to say so. Who did he think he was? Giving her permission!

"And who will pay for it, Sir?"

"Pay for it. Pay for it? Yes. Don't worry, Sister. I will make arrangements." Maj. Deepak said, as she hung up, miffed. He had tried to be soothing, despite knowing it was wasted on Nursing Supe, with whom he had regular battles. This time he was going to make sure he would win, and she would lose.

Corporate Social Responsibility was the new buzzword in Hospital Administration, trickled down from multinational companies that had extended their roots into India. Hospitals in the private sector were having to find creative ways to show their philanthropy. Just the fact that their business was on paper "not for profit" or that it involved caring for people was not good enough anymore. Adopting villages, conducting mass vaccinations, school health checkups, free eye camps, free cancer detection camps – the list of activities were increasing every day. Maj. Deepak with his years of Army service had a soft corner for Trauma care. If he was going to have to throw money down the drain, he wanted to be able to throw it where he liked.

Thus it was, that today, the medical care of Mr.Unknown could continue beyond initial resuscitation in Casualty. From CT scan he went to the operating room to have a Neurosurgical procedure in which blood clots within his skull that were pressing down on his brain were evacuated, the bleeding points controlled, and a large portion of his skull bone was taken off, thoroughly cleaned of all road dirt and bone chips, and buried in a pocket under the skin of his abdomen to keep it viable for subsequent replacement with plates and screws once it was clear that brain swelling had subsided.

After the operation he was shifted to Surgical ICU. Brain swelling inevitably accompanied a severe head injury. Over the next days it would be managed by placing the patient on a ventilator to assist breathing, and keep the blood CO_2 levels low, while additionally giving medicines to dry out the surplus fluid in the brain.

Unknown, as he continued to be called, came out of surgery barely recognizable. His head was swathed in bandages, his eyes covered with eye pads that concealed the hideous bruising seen in Casualty. An 'endotracheal tube' entered via his mouth into his trachea and lungs, and a 'nasogastric tube' emerged from one nostril draining his stomach. He had a 'central line' in his neck, giving a continuous read out, enabling estimation of pressures in the large veins on the right side of his heart. To measure blood pressure he had a pneumatic cuff wrapped around his arm. A bedside monitor periodically inflated the cuff and read out his blood pressure as a digital display. The amount of oxygen in his blood was estimated by a probe wrapped around a finger nail. It glowed red and lit up his finger-tip.

A nurse specially trained and experienced in high tech care took over from the anesthesiologist. She would look after him, continuously standing by his side, administering medications and iv fluids, watching the monitors, checking urine output, and periodically documenting the readings in an ICU chart that could be studied by Critical Care and Neurosurgery doctors for a detailed reconstruction of all preceding events that is critical to decision making. Every hour she turned him taking his weight off his back and protecting his skin from breaking down. Every hour she gave him chest physiotherapy thumping his chest and suctioning his endotracheal tube. She was always conscious that the life entrusted to her care hung by a thread. Everything could, and often did, change dramatically for better or worse during the course of her twelve hour shift.

It was hard work, but she loved it, constantly watching a dozen different parameters and keeping them all within the normal range. Anything drifting away from normal bothered her a great deal, and she would get on the phone to alert the doctors and make sure she got what she needed – new ideas, new investigations, a different strategy for the fluids and drugs, a specialist consultation – whatever it took to restore equilibrium to the *milieu interior*, the internal environment where cellular function took place. Where her patient's cells were clinging to life.

When her shift ended she wanted her patient to have a steady heart rate, stable blood pressure, good urine output, clear chest with a normal blood gas report (good oxygen and carbon dioxide levels, no imbalance in acid and base, normal lactic acid and bicarb levels), normal electrolytes (sodium, potassium, chloride, bicarb, calcium, phosphorus, and magnesium). That was her goal.

Surrounded by gadgets, she watched a stack of infusion pumps, the ventilator, transduced lines feeding into monitors overhead and by the side of the patient, ever alert to the alarms that would go off if anything malfunctioned or if something was wrong. More importantly, she watched her patient, trusting her instincts to tell her if something was not right, constantly watching for physical signs that might signal a subtle change that monitors might not pick up.

Like a runner in a relay race, straining to keep her place and perhaps surge ahead during her lap, she worked her shift with one goal: to hand over her patient to the nurse who came on the next shift in better shape than when she took charge. And when she could do so, it gave her work satisfaction like none other.

It did not matter to her whether the patient was known or Unknown, a President or a pauper. To her, every patient was a precious child whose very existence depended on her. It was hard not to get emotionally attached to a patient in this situation, and she knew it led to heartbreak if her patient died. Even so, she knew for a fact that a patient in such a critical life and death struggle could not survive unless she put her heart and soul into her job, never mind the consequences.

ICU nurses are a special breed.

The man in the background, up in the Administrative section of the hospital, making this massive rescue effort happen, remained as he liked to be: an invisible presence.

Maj. Deepak had always marched to his own drum. Born into a Malayalee family with rich Naval traditions he had chosen to join the Army and spend his military career in arid mountain ranges, desert landscapes, and lush sub Himalayan jungles of north India. An indifferent student in medical college he decided he had no interest in the usual rat race after graduation, struggling to find a residency in ever narrowing specialties to end up treating conditions that affected a minuscule segment of the population. He had used the Army to buy himself time, and the Army had shown him where his talent lay. After a few years in 'border postings' when sent to Lucknow for the mandatory course for all medical officers to revise the medicine they had forgotten, he had to everyone's surprise effortlessly topped the course. The Army brass, always looking for their next star, had asked him which medical or surgical specialty he would like, and he answered to their chagrin that none interested him. He wanted to go into Administration – usually the refuge of those who could not get anything 'better'.

Recently back in Kerala, after his years of 'short service' he was immediately in demand, with lucrative pay several multiples of his Army pension. Glad to have the pension to fall back on, apart from an old boys network of Administrators who could get him jobs overseas, he had decided he could take risks, and focus his talents on something that was the real need of the hour, even if not considered fashionable or lucrative.

Maj. Deepak wanted to be a leader. A leader, he had learned in the course of his business studies, had to be more than a mere manager. The difference was that a leader effected change. The Army with its rigid hierarchy had few if any leadership opportunities, and he had grown frustrated in the service. He could not wait to get out into the civilian world where the opportunities were much more. He began to look for where he could start.

Trauma care became his project first, his obsession later, and in time would be his legacy. Statistics from the around the world showed that Trauma had become the commonest cause of death in the age group of 15 to 45 years of age. Most hospital administrators he spoke with had a dread of it. Nobody wanted to do anything to try and solve the problem. They would recite the usual litany of high costs and the uncertainty of recovering them. Dealing with the judicial system was never any fun. After their strenuous work, in nearly every case doctors would have to run to court whenever summoned, as cases dragged on for years. Although in theory they were supposed to be expert witnesses, helping the court to make a judgment about how much compensation to award to an accident victim, lawyers for the vehicle owner and his insurance company would harass the doctor, trying to make it seem as though the disabilities were the result of faulty medical care and not the accident itself. The whole business was unpalatable.

Hoping for some elected government to fix the broken system by enacting new legislation was to dream the impossible. Even in the US, he was reminded, health care legislation was political suicide. Wherever in the world you looked, people on the take of easy insurance money were powerful, could easily buy political influence, and unwilling to let anyone cut in on their game.

The surgeons he spoke to, by and large, had no problem with looking after trauma victims. They just wanted to be paid for their work, and if possible not have to keep going to court while the compensation process wound its way through the judicial system.

Many hospitals had already solved this difficulty by having one designated senior Casualty Medical Officer who would handle all cases and depose in court working off the medical record. Surgeons rarely waste their time in court these days, waiting their turn in the witness stand.

Having studied the situation, he realized the problem was really quite straightforward:

- Most civilian trauma was caused by motor vehicles plying on public roads
- All vehicles had to be insured by their owners.
- There was, therefore, enough insurance money available for medical care of trauma victims
- This money was being disbursed through Tribunals and courts as "compensation". Calculating the amount of compensation was a convoluted process at the "Motor Accident Claims Tribunal" where rash and negligent behavior had to be proved and settlements were based on calculations of "disability" and "loss of income". Invariably, there was room for negotiation, and a nexus of insurance agents and lawyers had evolved around the lucrative business.

The key to the treasure was of course in the hands of lawyers "specializing" in accident cases. To get hold of it in a timely manner in order to pay for medical treatment of accident victims, he would have to seek their cooperation.

For the most part however, hospital administrators were too lazy to do what was needed. Some liked to play coy, "you don't want to be getting mixed up with ambulance chasers, do you?" they asked.

Maj. Deepak got his break through a senior police officer who was addicted to golf and always looking for a chance to play on the course available to Naval and Army officers at the Naval base in Kochi.

"How do you think these lawyers get their cases?" the police officer asked.

There were two ways. They could hang out outside hospitals and directly solicit their clients, or they could get the police who were involved in the case to direct a family member of the victim to them. For a small fee, of course.

Working through the golfer, Maj. Deepak found the lawyers in the area to whom vehicular trauma cases were being directed by the police. One by one he called them in for a discussion and gradually got an idea of how they worked, and what they needed to be effective. He knew that the first requisite of successful negotiation was to properly understand the other person's views and difficulties. Everybody had some need that required to be met, and some problem that they needed solved. Soon the elements of his plan began to take shape.

The first requirement was to appoint a "Trauma Coordinator". Maj Deepak looked for an ex-serviceman for this job. Calling up the Convenor of the ex-servicemen's union, he found half a dozen people who could fit the job description he had in mind, and soon found the right person.

Former Havildar Suresh Nambiar used to be an instructor at the Army School of Physical Training in Pune, and still looked the part with a fiercely curled moustache and the ample shoulders and belly of a powerlifter. His job would be to liase with ambulance drivers and police and determine the details of the accident, the vehicles involved, their insurance status, and all the information normally collected by the police as part of their investigation. Hav. Nambiar soon made friends with the key policemen in the local police station. An entire career dedicated to making senior Army officers comply with their drill and physical fitness requirement, had equipped Hav. Nambiar with the skills needed to talk to people above his rank, and bend them to his will. All those below him in rank were either terrified of him, or loved him – it didn't matter which because they would follow him to death anyway.

Working off a road map of the Kochi area, and police reports of accident statistics, Nambiar identified places in the vicinity where the most accident victims were likely to be encountered. He then sent his hospital public relations department personnel to go to each spot, and identify primary care providers, nursing homes and dispensaries in the neighborhood, to find out how often they saw accident victims and where they were then being referred. Local ambulance drivers were interviewed and slowly a pattern emerged. Word of mouth advertising was done to tell all the important people thus identified – Maj. Deepak called them "stakeholders" – about the facilities available at his center.

Everyone was happy to find that a senior hospital administrator in a well equipped hospital was willing to take on Trauma cases.

A succession of road accident victims began to be ferried to the Casualty. Their payments were made either by themselves when they could, or referred to the lawyers identified by Maj. Deepak to take their case to the Motor Accident Tribunal and file for a compensation amount that included the hospital bill. So called "ambulance chasers" were now an enthusiastic component of a Trauma response system.

It remained to be seen what would happen in a really major trauma case, where the vehicle involved was not identified – a "hit and run" case. The provision in law for such cases was unclear and the victim was left with only the minimum compensation provided under the law – a token amount that had not been revised for decades to reflect the actual sums of money required for medical care of any kind other than first-aid.

Mulling over possible solutions to this problem, Maj. Deepak realized that only an actual experience of such a case would help him formulate a plan of action. It was unknown territory and he knew he would have to step out into it, before he could chart a course for the future.

That was when Unknown had arrived, bleeding, unconscious, broken: a 'hit-and-run' case with no witnesses, and no family members on hand to pay any of the hospital expenses which were mounting by the minute.

Ayesha was almost ready to give up. Waiting for something is hard. Waiting with no idea how long the wait will be is the hardest thing to do.

And what were they waiting for? Sometimes it bothered her that they were really waiting for someone to die and donate their organs, and hoping the liver would match for Kunju.

She was now seeing a new side to her husband that she did not know existed. This was a strangely stronger side of him that had surfaced even as he was weakened by his illness and blood loss. He was never one to talk much, but now he had a kind of intensity, more focused, concentrating on something in his silences. To divert his mind he would watch the sports channel. Some years earlier, Raza had found him a set of videos on boxing and he would watch them whenever he had free time in the evenings. Although they were scratchy and of poor quality, he never tired of watching old match-ups from the '60s and '70s. Mohammed Ali, the boxer who overcame powerful opponents inside and outside the ring was his favorite.

Once, during one of his silences, when Ayesha asked him what he was thinking about he told her he had got a lawyer to draw up his will and he wanted her to look at it when it was ready. He told her that their house had already been registered as a joint ownership with her, and she should always keep it. All their savings and sources of income were listed in the will. She already knew about them, but had not been keeping up lately. She would have to learn about them now, and know the systems he had put in place to make sure they were managed properly.

That had frightened her. She was alone at home most of the time now, since Kunju had insisted that Raza and Shehnaz go back to college. Shehnaz would call every evening, and that was a source of comfort to both of them. After a few sentences with Kunju, Ayesha would take the phone and retreat to the bedroom, where mother and daughter could talk in peace. When she told Shehnaz about how gruesome it felt to be waiting for a donor, her daughter told her not to worry about it. People were dying every day. Many lives and organs were going waste all the time. Thank God some people donated their organs and could save the lives of others.

Both Shehnaz and Raza had signed donor cards. They had gone onto the website of KNOS, and got the information they needed.

It was not enough to sign a card, they learned, they had to inform their family members of their wish, since it was the family who would be taking the decision on their behalf.

Ayesha did not know whether she approved of this or not. She asked Kunju whether it was against their religion to donate organs after death. To her surprise, Kunju had a ready answer. He had looked up the matter and also consulted with an uncle of his who was the person in the family with the most knowledge about religious matters. A religious scholar, who also had a doctorate in mathematics, this uncle often spoke of how math, astronomy and other sciences had been nurtured and advanced from the very beginning by Islam. He was always a welcome guest at the Aliyar Kunju home and a fascinating conversationalist.

The highest council of Islamic scholars had approved organ donation and transplantation. Muslims regularly donated organs in Saudi Arabia, Iran, and in other Islamic and non-Islamic countries where they had transplant programs. In India this was just starting, and some confusion did exist, but the reality was that there was no religious objection to organ donation after death in any of the major world religions.

Kunju continued to work, though now he would leave later than his usual time to avoid the morning rush hour traffic. He rearranged his office and moved in a large reclining easy chair on which he could stretch out to sleep in the afternoon for an hour.

Every two weeks Ayesha would accompany Kunju to the Transplant Center.

He was feeling relatively well now, and usually there was no need to wait to see the doctors. The person they had to meet regularly was the Transplant Coordinator. The 'young man with the non-Malayalee accent' as they had first labeled him, now had a name – Rajeev. He had become their best friend. Rajeev would call to remind them of their clinic visits. They would go to the lab and get their blood tests done. Then there was a visit to the Nutrition department where Bhagyalaxmi, or one of her pretty juniors would check Kunju's weight, and do a diet recall with Ayesha. They had to make sure he was getting adequate protein and calories in his diet. Ayesha would often have questions based on what she had heard or read.

To Kunju's great relief the Nutritionist had not insisted he become vegetarian, even though this had been the discharge advice he had been given at the hospital where Mustafa had taken him when he first vomited blood. Restricting dietary intake of protein was necessary if some complications of liver disease had occurred, but not as a routine, and certainly not now while he was waiting for a transplant.

The Physiotherapy department visit usually followed. Kunju looked forward to this part of the visit. He had achieved all their targets for walking, lifting weights, and breathing exercises. He was planning to get a home gym set up and would discuss the various options available in the market with the physiotherapist he liked.

Running into Krish at the Physiotherapy department was always fun. Though a recent acquaintance, he was now like an old friend. This was a new experience for the normally reserved Kunju, and both he and Ayesha looked forward to meeting him. He continued to be his irrepressibly cheerful self, and they always felt energized afterwards.

They often had lunch together at the Hospital cafeteria. One day Krish was looking uncharacteristically depressed. They asked him how he was feeling, just to be polite, and found that he was in a mood to elaborate. In his usual extroverted way of holding back nothing personal, he described how he had been called in the previous night for a transplant, but the person just ahead of him on the list had got the kidney.

"Why would they call you in if they were not going to give you the kidney?" Ayesha wondered aloud.

"The other person was ahead of me on the list, but if he had not matched with the donor, I would have got the kidney. When the result came from the lab we had both matched, but he was ahead so it was his turn."

"Oh you must have felt so disappointed!" she cried.

"Yes, I was," said Krish quietly, "but at least I know now that I am on the top of the list in my blood group, and it may not be long before I get my chance."

He was smiling again, back to his usual self.

By afternoon Kunju's lab results would be in, and they would meet Rajeev who would give them a copy "for their records", he always said, along with the calculated MELD score. The MELD score would fluctuate a point or two up or down, and they would try to figure out what they may have done to make Kunju's condition better or worse. If they had a question, Rajeev would answer it, or call one of the doctors to discuss it with them.

Mustafa would invariably have some news for them when they were ready to return from hospital. They called it the Parking Lot news. Sometimes he would be talking about the dignitaries who had come to the hospital that day. He would know everything about which doctor they had come to see, and what the illness was or might be. Cancer had long been his favorite diagnosis, and he had always kept a look out for all actors or politicians likely to be secretly suffering from this 'emperor of maladies'. Now, of course, he was investigating transplantation, and was hoping to find out who had either received one, or was waiting for a transplant. He was not having much luck.

"Too bad none of our Chief Ministers has needed a transplant," he said with heated indignation. "Look at Tamil Nadu! Today I was talking to a Tamilian driver. He had brought a patient all the way from Coimbatore! It was amazing how much he knew about this Transplant business. All Tamilians know about transplant because MGR had a kidney transplant."

Mustafa was not happy that Kerala had fallen behind Tamil Nadu in this area.

"What did he tell you about transplant, Mustafa?" asked Kunju, encouraging him to talk despite getting a disapproving look from Ayesha.

"He couldn't tell me anything I did not already know," said Mustafa stoutly, ever the competitive Malayalee. "He knew nothing about liver transplant. Kidney, kidney, kidney! That's all he could talk about! I told him liver is much bigger than kidney. He kept quiet after that!"

Across town in the Trauma unit, the combined efforts of Maj. Deepak, and Hav. Nambiar had resulted in Unknown being identified. A Missing Person report had been filed from a small town on National Highway, 47, the day after Unknown had been admitted to hospital, and police investigations revealed that Unknown was actually Jose Avirachen from a suburb of Trichur.

Jose, 32 years old, was a small businessman running a bakery and its adjacent shop that sold 'English Medicines'. His wife Seleena who did not suspect anything was wrong till noon when she called him and got no answer, had filed the Missing Person report. She was shocked to hear that her husband was in hospital with a head injury after a serious road accident.

"How can it be?" she asked in disbelief, "he always wore a helmet".

Even as the words left her mouth, she realized that he had not worn his helmet that morning. In fact he had not taken his motorcycle to work as it had a flat tire, and he was late. She was in the kitchen when he yelled out that he would be taking the bus, and had actually been glad he was doing so, as she always worried when he rode his bike in chaotic traffic.

The safety associated with riding a big bus in Kerala is, however, often negated by the driving habits of the driver. With the backing of strong trade unions, bus and truck drivers in India regard themselves unfettered by rules that apply to lesser vehicles on the road. They stop where they will and often in the middle of the road, far from designated bus stops. Vehicles following the bus have to swerve to avoid the suddenly stalled behemoth in the middle of the road. It was at one such unexpected halt that Jose had realized he was close to the shop of one of his suppliers, and might be able to meet him and close a deal. He had jumped up from his seat, and rushed to the door, managing to get out just as the bus got moving again. He landed in the middle of the road and in the path of a car desperately trying to catch up with vehicles that had managed to get past the bus.

He never saw what hit him from behind, and was soon airborne as the low front fender hit his legs, lifting him off his feet. His head hit the top of the windshield where it meets the metal, and he was immediately and mercifully rendered unconscious as his body rolled over the roof and off the side like a rag doll. He did not cry out, and there was no sound. The only eye witness was a young boy. Nobody had taken notice of the car or its license plate as it sped away.

A passing autorickshaw with three passengers in it stopped. The driver wanted to take Jose to the nearest hospital. An argument had ensued, the passengers more keen to go on, and the auto driver asking them to get off and help him load Jose into the back seat. The exchange soon got heated, with the auto driver threatening to reduce the passengers to the same condition as the figure on the roadside if they did not get out and help. One of the passengers, a devotee of non-violent principles in life, had quickly called the Rotary club ambulance from his cell phone, and ended the argument.

At the Trauma center, Seleena had difficulty identifying the bandaged and blackeyed individual with the tubes coming out of his mouth and nose as her husband. The policeman waiting impatiently for her signature on some papers had made her so nervous she could not even think. Her signatures never came out the same twice, and she had never signed a police document before. With a shaking hand she scribbled her name on the paper, not caring to read what she was signing. The nurse looking after Jose appeared hostile at first, blaming Seleena's late arrival for many of the difficulties she had been facing with procuring medicines and getting consent for various procedures. Fortunately the shift changed, and the night nurse was much more willing to explain things and also to comfort Seleena. Jose's parents were the next to arrive, and they were of course only an extra burden for Seleena with their millions of questions, many of which were with the intention of trying to fix blame for what had happened. As though it was all her fault!

After her initial shock at the hospital bill that was presented to her, Seleena was actually grateful as it transferred the ire of her in-laws to the hospital authorities, and the "unnecessary stuff" they were doing. The bill was already close to exceeding the dowry she had brought when she got married to Jose 3 years ago. There was of course no way she could afford to pay it. They did not have that kind of money saved, and no, they did not have any medical insurance, Seleena was perversely pleased to inform the nosy Nursing Supervisor who had come to interview them in the ICU waiting area.

When Maj. Deepak was informed by Nursing Supe that Unknown, who she still refused to refer to by his real name, was not likely to have his expenses met, he had to think fast.

"Don't worry, Sister", he had bluffed, "I have our social services working on it."

The Social work department in the hospital comprised two very voluble ladies with staunchly liberal political views, and their silenced department chief who was politically confused. He had started out liberal and was now leaning to becoming conservative. He knew from bitter experience the futility of social work that was not backed by considerable "money power", as he liked to refer to that imaginary mother lode of wealth located someplace inaccessible to ordinary mortals like himself.

Of the many possible functions for a social worker in a hospital, the one most often utilized was their socio-economic function. In fact, some doctors and nurses thought they were there solely to help the hospital recover expenses from parsimonious patients. Intensive care units, where cost overruns were common, were consequently an area of the hospital constantly contacting Social Services for help. ICUs also generated the maximum number of complaints by patients and their families, and dissatisfaction, everyone knew, is often the starting point for litigation. Social workers had to step into conflicts and try to resolve them. They were the ones working with the patient's family while doctors and nurses worked on the patient.

Maj. Deepak, who tended to also use social workers as his eyes and ears for what was happening around the hospital, enjoyed his interactions with his social workers. He called them his "MSWs" but thought of them as his KGB, although Renita middle aged and grumpy, and Sunita, young fresh and cheerful, hardly fit the profile of secret service agents. He now summoned Sunita and assigned the case to her.

Although Maj. Deepak had not considered Sunita to have any special skills or training for the particular case he had assigned to her, the fact was that she had worked in the famous Sri Chitra Tirunal neuroscience center in Trivandrum, and had experience of working with patients like Unknown alias Jose Avirachen. She was overjoyed to be asked to manage this case.

While in Sri Chitra, she had seen plenty of patients in coma, and was aware of how traumatic this could be for family members who would have lots of questions regarding the possibility of recovery and whether their patient, so obviously disabled, would ever be normal again.

She also knew how difficult it is for doctors to be sure of the outcome in such cases. They were busy trying to save life, and a live person was often their major goal. However, with the severe deficiency of good rehabilitation services, and home nursing that was usually unskilled, a patient with severe neurological impairment was difficult to look after once he or she had survived intensive care. There were no long term nursing homes, specific for the needs of these patients, and the few that provided basic generalized long term care were expensive and beyond the reach of most people.

Seeking answers to questions for which no ready answers were available in Trivandrum, she had looked at other institutions for extra training. She had visited the Apollo hospital in Chennai, NIMHANS (National Institute for mental health and neurosciences) in Bangalore, and CMC (Christian Medical College) in Vellore. Gradually, a picture had formed in her mind about how to approach this difficult situation from a social work point of view, with her focus on the families of neurologically impaired patients.

Quickly going down to the ICU where Jose Avirachen was admitted, she found out all she could from talking to the nurses looking after him and from studying the chart and doctors' notes. She made it a point to be present at the bedside when the doctors did their rounds. She studied the bedside chart, and spoke with the nurses looking after the patient. She realized that the patient's "GCS" (Glasgow Coma Score) was 8 on admission. She recalled how critical it was to explain to family members what the GCS was, and how the Neurosurgeons and nurses monitored the GCS. She noted that the GCS had not improved after the operation performed by the Neurosurgeons to remove blood clots and stop bleeding in his brain. The outlook did not seem very good. This poor patient's family would have a lot to deal with, she knew.

The next morning, when Hav. Nambiar, the Trauma Coordinator, informed her that Unknown had been identified, and his family had been contacted, she rushed to the surgical ICU to meet them. Her training was, first and foremost, to identify the "Power Person" in the family.

Every family is unique, and the person wielding the maximum influence when it came to decision making, was the one referred to as the Power Person ("PP"). Very often, the breadwinner in the family is the PP, but this could vary from one family to another. In Kerala, unlike other states in India, Sunita was aware that the PP was often a female in the family. Sometimes it was an uncle or aunt who had the most education. Very often a distant person, either in India or abroad, or a religious figure outside the family would be consulted by the family when it came to important decisions. Religious figures, Sunita knew, could be particularly difficult if they did not understand medical realities, and would speak from the point of view of faith, or social customs that masquerade as religion. She knew that the concept of autonomy in medical decision making was unusual in India where patients usually allow doctors to make decisions for them, instead of stating their wishes regarding the medical measures being taken. Patients, she knew, rarely actually read the Consent Forms they signed.

Inside Neuro ICU she first went to the nurse looking after Jose, and found out that there had been no improvement in his condition overnight. He used to be breathing at a rate of between 20 and 30 breaths per minute, but now was down to hardly breathing at all, totally dependent on the ventilator to breathe for him. There was no response to pain indicating a very deep level of coma. His eyes were fixed and staring when they took off his eye pads which were necessary to protect his eyes as he was not blinking his eyelids at all and required protection to prevent corneal abrasions. When shining a torchlight into his eyes, the nurse had noted that unlike yesterday when he still had some reaction to light, today his pupils were not reacting at all.

"Do you think he is brain dead?" Sunita asked the ICU nurse.

"I don't know. I don't think so, because he still moves when I suction his throat and I feel he tenses his muscles a little when I move him from side to side to bathe him and do skin care."

"OK. I believe the family members have arrived. Did you meet any of them?"

"Yes, they are sitting there in the waiting room. And no, I did not meet any of them. I have my hands full with looking after their patient, and rounds will be starting soon."

Sunita recognized the "I am too busy to bother with the family – that's your work" message in the ICU nurse's voice. She decided to meet the family before doctors' rounds.

In the waiting room the new family was easy to identify. Sunita went over to them and introduced herself, giving them the usual line that she was there for them and they should feel free to ask her for any required help. The older man and woman, who Sunita later found out were Jose's parents did not seem to connect with her, but the younger woman, introduced herself as the patient's wife, and appeared interested in what Sunita had to offer. It became clear that this was the person who would most likely be taking the tough decisions. Sunita was happy with this situation, because the wife is the first legal "next-of-kin", and would be the one to approach for all matters concerning the patient.

Sunita soon found out that Seleena and Jose had two young children, who she had left with a neighbor when she came to the hospital. The older girl was 8 and the younger boy was 3 years old. The children were alone at home. She could gather that Seleena trusted her daughter to look after her younger brother. A neighbor had promised to keep an eye on them. There was a phone at home by which she could communicate with the children when needed. Jose's parents were clearly not an integral part of her daily life or support system.

Seleena was actually more keen to make an international call to her brother who was in Dubai, and inform him about what had happened. Sunita took her over to her office where she had international dialing privileges, and helped Seleena place the call. Overhearing her talk to her brother she quickly realized her initial assessment was correct as to who the power person was in this family.

The call over, they headed back to the waiting area, and Sunita promised to come back and explain things to her after rounds, and also to arrange a meeting between the Neurosurgeon and the family.

Inside the ICU, rounds did not take long. Completing his examination of Jose, the Neurosurgeon said this looked like a hopeless case, and in his opinion the patient was brain dead or soon would be. The matter had to be explained to the patient's family as soon as possible. He had an operation to do, and had to be going into the Operation Theater soon.

Sunita brought Jose's family to the Conference room next to the ICU and had them sit down while waiting for the Neurosurgeon. When he came in he had already changed into his OT clothes and wore a cap with his mask dangling around his neck.

Sunita introduced Seleena first, and Jose's parents next, the emphasis in her introductions indicating to the Neurosurgeon who he should be primarily focused on. He didn't pay much attention to Sunita, eager to get on with what he had to say. He spoke to the family as a whole, eyes flitting from one person to the other.

"Your patient arrived here in a very serious condition. His GCS was 8, and this tells us how seriously the brain is injured. We had to operate as an emergency, but this morning his GCS score has dropped to 3. I think he is very serious and there is a good chance he may not survive."

Sunita was watching the family members closely while the Neurosurgeon was speaking. While Jose's mother seemed to break down, and his father looked confused, she could see that Seleena was alert and paying close attention.

"What does this score mean, Sir?" she asked, "is this something you see on the brain scan? What does his scan report show?"

The Neurosurgeon looked impatiently at his watch.

"I have an operation that I have to start soon. I will have to find some time afterwards to explain everything to you."

Sunita decided to step in.

"I can start explaining things to the family in a general sense, Sir, and they will be better able to have this discussion when you are free," she offered.

"OK. Ask the nurse to explain the present condition. If there are any doubts, I should be free in about 4 hours." And with that he left.

Sunita knew she would have a lot of work, but this was what she enjoyed – explaining medical details to patients' family members in a layperson's words, using terms that they could easily understand. She thought she could do a good job, and anyway doctors and nurses were too busy.

Not being a doctor or a nurse, was actually an advantage to Sunita, as people related to her more easily, and did not feel intimidated as they might when talking to someone with the advantage of many years of medical training, and a much better understanding of things than they could ever hope to have.

A large part of education, Sunita knew, lay in the confidence that a teacher inspires in the student.

She had noted the fact that Seleena was asking the questions, and had asked what the scan reports were. Hospital policy was to give copies of all reports to the patients if asked, so she could get duplicates of the reports for Seleena. This would give her the opportunity she needed to gain the confidence of Jose's family.

Asking the family to stay in the Conference room she went back to her office to photocopy the scan reports and also to fetch an atlas of brain anatomy with illustrations that she had found useful when she had to explain things to patients when working in Sri Chitra. She would use the atlases to explain the scan reports if needed. Carefully she went over in her mind the interaction between the family and the Neurosurgeon. The first question she would have to address was about the GCS scoring system which she remembered Seleena asking.

In the 1960s and early '70s, a simple scoring system had been developed in Glasgow, Scotland, to evaluate someone who was in a coma following head injury. Three responses were noted:

1. Eyes: What were the eyes doing? Was the person looking around at what was happening around him? Or were the eyes not seeing anything, not moving in response to being called or when the head was moved?

2. Verbal: Was the speech normal? Did the person answer coherently and did he know who he is, also where, and what day or time it is? Or was there only incoherent crying or mumbling, or no speech at all?

3. Motor movements: This was usually tested with the administration of a slightly painful stimulus such as pressing on the nail to see what the patient would do. Was he capable of accurately identifying the pain and removing his hand? Or did it set off some abnormal spasms? (see appendix 1 for details)

Each response was given a score from 1 to 5. The maximum score was 15 and signified an essentially fully conscious individual. The minimum score was 3, and indicated deep coma.

The scoring system had quickly become popular worldwide and made Bryan Jennett, and Graham Teasdale, the Scottish Neurosurgeons in Glasgow who had published it in 1974, world famous. Called the Glasgow Coma Score, or GCS, it could be quickly calculated at the accident site where rescuers had found the injured person, and afterwards all along the course of treatment. It gave a degree of objectivity to the assessment of coma.

The scoring system for coma was quickly adopted in wars from Falklands to Iraq, from Sierra Leone to Sri Lanka, and in civilian traumatic brain injury all over the world. In countries with advanced roadside rescue systems in place, the GCS along with blood pressure became the two most important pieces of information relayed to the hospital from the field as the Trauma team in the hospital got ready for a patient being rushed in by ambulance. Everyone from Emergency medical technicians, nurses and doctors used the GCS to understand each other and to record the progress of a patient with head injury.

In the half century that had gone by since the GCS was developed, all kinds of advanced techniques had been developed to study the brain: CT scans, MRI scans, Nuclear medicine brain perfusion scans, intracranial and intraventricular pressure monitoring, and the list promised to keep growing. Nothing had been able to replace the simple GCS which had repeatedly proved its value at bedside and streetside for making an assessment of how the brain was working.

In Jose Avirachen's case, the GCS on arrival had been 8. That meant that out of a possible highest score of 15 he had a score of only 8. This immediately put the severity of his brain injury very high, and he qualified to be categorized as a "catastrophic brain injury".

After resuscitation in the Casualty he had made no improvement in his GCS, and the score had continued to be 8 when he returned from the Operation Theater. The outlook was bleak.

The next day his GCS had deteriorated further to 3, and this was the situation when his family first saw him. His chances of survival had worsened to nearly zero.

The human brain is a jelly like structure full of delicate nerves and their connecting fibers. Severe injury caused by sudden movement of the head resulted in movement of the brain within the skull. Areas of different density moved at different speeds, and resulted in shearing forces that disrupted fragile connections within the brain.

Nerve connections once torn apart rarely connect properly again. It is analogous to cutting across an electric cord, and then trying to reconnect the two ends by correctly aligning each individual strand of the wire so that the original is restored intact.

At the two ends of each nerve strand are the nerve cells communicating with each other via the strand. If the blood supply to these is cut off, as commonly happens when the brain swells, then the entire delicate structure is irreversibly damaged.

The human brain has been called the most complex computer ever designed. It doesn't take much to destroy the mother board. The most complex part of a computer is also its most delicate.

Primary injury to the brain was something that could not be reversed by surgery or medications. The only hope was to keep the patient alive by optimizing the function of all the other organs; restrict injury to the delicate brain by correcting blood pressure and giving oxygen; and operating early if blood collections within the skull were pressing on the brain and making the primary injury worse.

Areas of the brain that were damaged at the very first instant, that millisecond when the head hits the road, or a bullet enters the brain, are usually gone forever. Nothing can be done to recover or revive the structures damaged by the primary injury.

If however the primary injury can be limited by early intervention like rapid rescue and resuscitation, efficient management of blood pressure and blood flow to the brain, and good oxygen delivery by skillful management of the airway and breathing, and timely neurosurgical intervention to stop bleeding within the brain and decompress collections of blood within the skull that put pressure on the brain itself, then there is a chance of survival.

Later treatment would be directed at rehabilitation and would depend on the phenomenon called 'neuroplasticity': the recently recognized possibility for uninjured regions of the brain being able to gradually take over function of the areas that were irreversibly destroyed. This was, naturally more likely to happen in children than in adults.

Everyone knows how difficult it is to teach an adult anything new.

That's a 'no brainer' chuckled Sunita to herself as she refreshed her memory about the topics she would have to talk about to the family of Unknown alias Jose Avirachen lying in the ICU with his head smashed.

The ultimate outcome of a "Traumatic Brain Injury" patient could be predicted to some extent by the GCS at the time of the injury, and also by the way the GCS either improved or worsened with time and treatment.

At this time, Sunita knew, Jose's chances of reaching the last phase of care i.e., the Rehabilitation Center appeared remote. It was much more likely that he was going to die. She struggled with how she would break the news to his young wife.

On returning to the ICU waiting area, Sunita found that Jose's parents had gone home. Apparently his father who was in his sixties, was convinced that if he did not have his meals exactly on time, three times daily, a national calamity with catastrophic global ramifications would occur. Along with several fastidious dietary restrictions and particularities, the whole process of food production and consumption in the senior Avirachen home had taken on the complexity and countenance of a United Nations exercise. Much thought, discussion, search, research, and combined action was necessary for constant culinary activity that world peace might prevail. Seleena was sitting alone. There were other patients' families in the waiting area. Knowing how intensely inquisitive her Malayali community is, Sunita took Seleena over to the Conference Room where they would have some privacy.

She soon realized that Seleena was very brave, very strong, and had a clear head despite her grief. She looked at the scan reports and asked for explanations which Sunita gave, explaining the concept of GCS, and also the kind of operation performed to relieve pressure on the brain from a blood clot forming inside his skull. She also said that despite this, the GCS had not improved, and had actually deteriorated to the lowest score possible.

"Will he recover to normal?" Seleena asked.

Sunita realized that this was difficult question for her to answer.

"We will have to ask the Neurosurgeon this question, as I am not qualified to answer it," said Sunita.

"My brother just called me on my cell phone. He has asked me to fax these reports to him," said Seleena. "He has a good friend who is a doctor, who has promised to show the reports to his Neurosurgical colleagues."

The two women continued to talk, with Seleena becoming more comfortable with the Social Worker. Sunita learned that for a short time Seleena had considered a nursing career, but had dropped this plan when she got married. She had, however completed the necessary courses to be able to apply for admission to Nursing College, and this had actually made it easier for her to understand what was going on. She was concerned about the mounting hospital expenses, but was willing to think of this in terms of the outcome he would have, knowing that any expense was justified if the anticipated outcome was going to be good.

Unfortunately, that was not likely, and Sunita noted that Seleena had begun to think of, and perhaps accept that possibility already.

Sunita was adept at recognizing the different phases of grief. The first was usually 'Denial', when the person faced with bad news refused to accept it. Sometimes they would refuse to accept death had occurred in a loved one.

Sunita knew of several cases, some highly publicized, of people who would keep a dead body at home waiting for the person to wake up, unable to accept reality even when putrefaction had set in. The phase of 'Acceptance' was a good sign that grief had not caused a person to become unhinged, and was the first step to eventual recovery.

While the Neurosurgeon was busy with his case in the Operation Theater an important change had taken place in Jose's condition.

His nurse had found that he had suddenly begun to pour out urine. From a more or less steady rate of 60 to 70 cc per hour, it had jumped to 350 cc, and then to 500 cc per hour. The Critical Care Medicine specialist was informed, and he diagnosed "diabetes insipidus".

This was a serious complication in the context of a head injury with brain swelling.

The pituitary gland is located at the base of the brain, and controls many of the hormone functions of the body. It also secretes a hormone called vasopressin which maintains blood pressure, and conserves water in the body. What had happened to Jose was that this hormone had suddenly stopped being produced by the pituitary, and his kidneys had consequently lost the ability to conserve water.

Increase in urine production, normally a good sign, was an ominous development in this situation.

If immediate action was not taken, Jose's body would soon become dry, his blood sodium and chloride levels would rise dangerously and all his cells would be surrounded by highly salty water. Shipwrecked sailors, surrounded by sea water, are warned not to drink it because the salt would enter their blood and they would die. Jose's cells were in a similar situation. Surrounded by highly concentrated, 'hypertonic' saltwater, they would lose precious intra cellular fluid, shrivel up and die.

Diabetes insipidus is regarded by many as a fatal development. It is certainly a game changer. Suddenly, from one hour to the next, the entire approach to managing the patient has to change.

After a head injury, Neurosurgeons like to restrict iv fluids in order to prevent swelling of the brain. When Diabetes insipidus sets in, continuing the same policy can result in a drop in blood pressure, and poor circulation affecting the function of all organs, and death from multi-organ failure becomes imminent if swift and strenuous corrective action is not taken.

Neurosurgeons are busy surgeons because their skills are hard to master, and there are not too many of them around. Some are control freaks, determined that every single aspect of their patient's care be under their singular control. Others realize they cannot possibly do everything and focus on what they do best, leaving the rest to others. Critical Care Medicine (CCM) specialists or Intensivists are the doctors who specialize in management of patients in the ICU, and bring to the patient's bedside a wide range of skills, and the speed required for simultaneous management of multiple organ systems. Such holistic care of ICU patients where the situation can change perilously from one hour to the next, has, along with specialized Intensive Care Nursing, provided hope of survival for critically ill patients.

When Sunita checked in at the ICU after lunch, she saw a flurry of activity around Jose's bed. The CCM specialist and one assistant were setting up an arterial pressure monitoring system that would display his blood pressure as a continuous read-out on the overhead monitor and also enable frequent and rapid checking of blood samples on the ICU 'blood gas machine' for instant readings of oxygen, carbon dioxide, and electrolyte levels. Although this is considered standard of care for patients who are on a ventilator, in Jose's case the Neurosurgeon had decided to manage without it so far in order, perhaps, to reduce costs.

Sunita went to the ICU waiting area to look for Seleena and apprise her of the latest developments. She knew she would now have to start preparing Seleena for bad news.

"How is he doing?" was Seleena's first question.

"They are putting in an arterial pressure monitoring system to better monitor him," replied Sunita, carefully.

"Why? Is his blood pressure dropping?" asked Seleena.

"They have made a diagnosis of 'diabetes insipidus'. This means his urine output has increased a lot, and they need a constant and accurate read out of his blood pressure. That is of course not possible with the old machine, that needs a cuff on the arm being periodically inflated. This is much more efficient and it's what ICUs are meant to do," replied Sunita.

"Is this going to increase the cost of the treatment? A little while ago the nurse came and gave me the bill that is outstanding, and asked me to go and pay it. There is no way I can pay such a large amount of money right now. I just do not have it!" Seleena was barely able to control a sob.

Sunita put her arm around the distraught wife. They sat together in silence for a while.

"Don't worry about it now," she said reassuringly, although she had no solution for the financial problem, "we will find a way."

The other person who was concerned about escalating treatment costs was the Neurosurgeon when he emerged from the Operation Theater. He summoned the Critical Care specialist and they got into an argument. The ICU nurse was glad the patient's family members could not witness the unseemly quarrel or hear the angry words exchanged. The Neurosurgeon wanted to allow Jose to die by gradually de-intensifying treatment and allowing all his organs to fail. This was what he always did. The Critical Care specialist said he was welcome to do as he pleased, but putting in the arterial pressure monitoring system was the proper way to look after the patient until or unless the family decided they did not want any more treatment.

"Who will pay the bill?" the Neurosurgeon wanted to know.

The Critical Care specialist shrugged his shoulders. That was not his concern, he said, as he had often said before. Worrying about who will pay for the cost of treatment was not conducive to good medical decision making, as far as he was concerned. There were people in the Finance section of the hospital drawing good salaries who were being paid to worry about stuff like this. His job was to look after the patient well, that was what he had done, and that was what he planned to continue doing.

Before long, the matter had landed on the desk of Maj. Deepak. The Finance Secretary of the hospital stood before him. In his hand was a ream of computer printing paper covered with numbers in columns and rows.

"Unknown patient's bill, Sar," he announced in a sing-song voice, adding somewhat unnecessarily, "increasing only, Sar."

"Bill!" said Maj. Deepak, echoing the strain of a tune he often heard. He had no ready contrapuntal response in this instance, and did not want to say too much anyway. He had learned, over the years, not to add a chorus to his finance employees' chant.

"Bill," he repeated, more reflectively, considering the options.

Then, in a flash of bureaucratic inspiration he said, "We will deal with this issue tomorrow. For now we will continue to do everything that is necessary and medically indicated".

His voice was sonorous, and his words were just what the finance secretary wanted to hear. "Tomorrow and tomorrow and tomorrow" were the finance secretary's favorite Shakespearean quote. Although secretly overjoyed, he did not immediately budge, desirous in some kind of non-violent, Gandhian way to convey the immediacy and importance of his bill collecting duties.

Maj. Deepak eyed him sternly gathering up his brief case in order to leave. Faced with the frontally advancing Major, the finance secretary stepped meekly aside. He was not so sure Nursing Supe, who had egged him on to approach the Major, would have done the same, but he would leave that to tomorrow, and tomorrow, to deal with.

Overnight, Unknown, alias Jose Avirachen, died. His coma, persistent and deep, progressed to brain death.

The first person to suspect it was the ICU nurse looking after him in the night. She had noticed that he stopped responding by coughing as he usually did when she suctioned his breathing tube. His eyes persisted in the fixed stare, and his pupils dilated some more. She informed the duty doctor, a junior who was 'first-on-call', who in turn called the Critical Care Medicine consultant at home.

"Prepare for testing," came the order over the phone. "It is about midnight now so stop all medicines that might be causing sedation, and make sure his body temperature is not low. Send all his blood tests by 4 AM so we have everything in by 6 AM when I will come to examine the patient. We will do the Apnea Test after I examine him. Call the Neurosurgeon and tell him we will be testing at 7 AM if he wants to come. Call me immediately if his blood pressure or heart rate become abnormal."

The night duty doctor who had never done the testing for brain death was excited and eager to learn. This was not something you did every day, and you never knew when such an opportunity would come again.

However, an unprecedented problem occurred. The Neurosurgeon refused to allow the testing.

The Critical Care specialist had anticipated it, as they had earlier had disagreements on this issue. He would want to test for brain death and the Neurosurgeon would refuse to do so, taking the position that there was no need to diagnose brain death and all they had to do was to de-intensify the ICU care, and allow all organs to fail as they invariably did in a few hours or days.

The CCM specialist's stand was, if the Neurosurgeon was so keen to reduce the patient's bill why did he never waive his operating fee and ask the hospital to forego the operation related expenses? Why were intensive care related expenses considered unnecessary or excessive? This was, after all a classic case of "operation successful, but patient dead".

The night duty doctor, being junior and only interested in moonlighting between exams, was caught in the cross-fire of a battle he knew nothing about. When he called the CCM specialist back and said the neurosurgeon had forbidden him to proceed with the arrangements for brain death testing, he was ordered loudly to call the Senior General Manager and discuss the issue.

"Let him tell us what the hospital wants. I am fed up with this Neurosurgeon," stormed the CCM specialist over the phone. "I refuse to keep ventilating a dead body, and I do not agree with the policy to let the organs fail while the hospital collects ICU charges, and the Neurosurgeon collects his daily consultation fees on useless rounds while we continue this futile work. Let the Administration tell me what is their policy in such patients!"

The night duty doctor now knew he had no chance of getting any sleep that night. He was however secretly happy with the way the excitement was building, and with no hesitation picked up the phone to continue the battle.

Maj. Deepak woke up with his cell phone ringing at his bedside. His wife also woke, but pretended to be asleep so she could overhear the conversation without his knowing she was eavesdropping.

"Good evening, Sir," came the voice over the phone. "Actually, I should say 'Good Morning, Sir'. I am the night duty doctor speaking, Sir."

The plethora of salutations correcting for chronology in the middle of the night only served to further befuddle the retired Army doctor who had all his life slept a minimum of eight hours, as recommended in all preventive medicine texts, and had not been routinely required to think at 2 in the morning.

"Good night. Morning. I mean 'Good morning'. Night duty doctor. Yes," Maj. Deepak's conditioned reflexes of speech-thought were still functional at the unearthly hour.

His wife turned her back to her husband, barely suppressing a groan at the way the conversation was going. She hoped it would not go further downhill from this point on.

"Sir, I am calling about the head injury patient in the ICU, Sir," the night duty doctor was really laying on the salutations, "Unknown, Sir. Now known. Avirachen Jose, Sir."

Despite the junior doctor confusing the heck out of the patient's ID, Maj. Deepak immediately knew who he was talking about.

"Yeah, what about him?" he asked impatiently.

"He is brain dead, Sir!"

"Brain dead! Brain dead. Brain dead? How do you know that?," said Maj. Deepak. His wife kept her back turned, but slowly and surreptitiously turned her head back to bring both ears into service. This was getting interesting.

"Sir, I don't know, Sir. But, er, CCM specialist-sir wants to do the testing in the morning, Sir."

"Testing. Yes. Testing is good. So do the testing. Why are you calling me?" somewhat testily.

"Sir, but the Neurosurgeon-sir is saying no, he will not allow it, Sir." Night duty doctor could barely suppress the note of enjoyment that had crept into his voice.

"Not allow it. Not allow it? No. Why?" the fog was clearing in Maj. Deepak's brain.

"Sir, I don't know why, Sir. That is why I am calling you, Sir. CCM specialist-sir told to do what you say Sir."

"'What You say? You mean what I say? Yes. What do I say? Hmm," and after a pause, "I say, we should do the testing."

Maj. Deepak had reverted to another time-honored reflex he had learned in the fauj. Do something. When the choice is between doing nothing and doing something, do something.

"Yes Sir. Thank you, Sir. I will tell them, Sir." This time the night duty doctor was not afraid to let the enjoyment come through in his voice as he hung up.

Maj. Deepak sighed audibly, and lay back, ready to drift off to sleep again. He had a talent for sleep. 'Able to sleep the moment my head hits the pillow', he liked to say when proudly describing this natural ability.

His wife, however, had no such talent. Once awake she would take a long time to sleep again. As she lay mulling over what she had heard, she was irritated by the loud snore that came from the other side of the bed, and then as the cadence grew to a crescendo, irritation gave way to anger.

Turning over, she shook Maj. Deepak awake.

"Good night. No sorry, Good Morning," he mumbled incoherently.

"Wake up. Its me."

"Me. Yes, it's you," acknowledged the soporific Major, summoning whatever gallantry he could to this new and unexpected attack.

"What was this going on about somebody being Brain Dead?"

"Unknown. He's brain dead" explained Maj. Deepak as succinctly as he could.

"What on earth are you talking about?" his wife was getting shrill. "Will you please wake up and explain to me what is going on?"

"Explain. Yes," said Maj. Deepak. Somewhere a small voice in his head seemed to say that he owed no explanations about this to anybody, least of all to his wife. But he stilled the voice immediately. He was talking to his

'Colonel' as he referred to his wife. This too was part of Army etiquette. The wife was always granted one rank (honorary, of course) above the officer.

He sat up in bed, and recounted the story to his wife as best as he could remember all the facts about Unknown, alias Jose Avirachen.

"You need to go to the hospital now," said Mrs. (Colonel) Deepak. "Now" she repeated, before her husband got his chance to repeat what she said, as she knew he would.

"OK. But may I ask why? What am I supposed to do there at this time?" protested Maj. Deepak after his initial acceptance of the order to mobilize.

"Why? You are asking me why?" his wife was also a master at the art of dishing out conversation repeats, but with a more salty flavor.

"No… Yes. Why?"

"Because this is a serious matter. And your numbskull of a Neurosurgeon and your idiotic CCM specialist are having a fight over it and don't seem to get it into their thick heads that this Brain death business is a serious matter. That's why. If you go there, they will come running with their little tails between their legs, and they will do what needs to be done."

No order could have been more clearly issued or more clearly received. Maj. Deepak got out, got dressed, and was driving to the hospital within half an hour. He called ahead to tell the Night Duty doctor ("Sir, yes Sir!") to be ready for him in the ICU, and to invite the feuding specialists to come as well.

He had never done testing for brain death, and would have to read up on the subject. He would have to go by his office, and look up the procedure before going to the ICU. He could not remember the last time he had done any studying at 2 in the morning.

Brain death is a new term but it is not a new concept. From time immemorial the seat of life has been recognized as being somewhere inside the skull where the brain resides. The most critical vital senses are located in the head and neck. Decapitation was the surest way to end a life, and was the principal method of execution throughout the world until recent times.

Perhaps the first record of an attempt to define and diagnose death can be traced back to the account in the Brihadaranyaka Upanishad, the ancient and sacred book of Vedic knowledge. The teaching (IV4.1-6) was that death is recognized first by unconsciousness, and then the loss of different functions of the brain. In specific order, the Upanishad describes the loss of functions mediated by the twelve cranial nerves supplying the nose (cranial nerve I), eyes (cranial nerves II, III, IV, and VI), ears (cranial nerve VIII), touch, (Cranial nerve V), speech and tongue (IX, X, XI and XII), and finally the loss of the ability to breathe (see Appendix 2).

With startling clarity comes the concluding statement, *"The life breath leaves, with all other vital forces..."* Loss of the ability to breathe is the ultimate and final sign of the end of life, according to the Upanishad.

The need to define and diagnose brain death in modern times became necessary because of the increasing ability of the medical community to resuscitate people with no respiration, heartbeat or other external signs of life. Resuscitation from a near death state resulted in dramatic rescues, but this did not happen always, and soon it became apparent that in a significant percentage of cases resuscitation of the heart beat was possible, but merely postponed death. These were usually individuals who remained deeply comatose even after the heart beat was recovered. Ventilators were able to take over respiration, but prolonged ventilation in someone who was in an irreversible coma with no outcome other than gradual loss of all organ function, was recognized as futile.

In 1968 a committee at the Harvard Medical School in the US published a set of criteria whereby it became possible to diagnose brain death in such deeply comatose persons. The tests to be done to make this determination bear an uncanny resemblance to the criteria described centuries earlier in the Upanishad. All cranial nerves had to be tested, and when the parts of the brain connected to those nerves were found to have no function, the final test was the "Apnea Test". This involved actually disconnecting the ventilator and seeing if the comatose individual could breathe on his own. If he could not, brain death was diagnosed. For good measure all the tests were repeated after 4 to 6 hours, and confirmed. In the fifty-odd odd years since the Harvard criteria were published they had been repeatedly validated, and most countries had signed them into law.

Subsequently, complicated techniques were developed to diagnose brain death, including angiograms of the brain, and nuclear medicine scans. These were designed to demonstrate complete cessation of blood circulation in the brain, and some doctors insisted on doing these tests.

Diagnosing brain gangrene was more palatable than diagnosing 'brain death'.

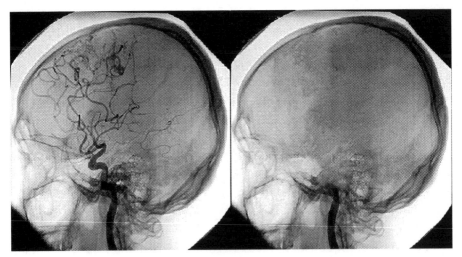

Brain death

Fig 3: Brain death. These two pictures showing the upper part of the neck and the head, are taken during angiogram of the brain. On the left side is the picture of a normal brain. The contrast dye injected into the carotid artery, seen in the neck as a black tubular structure, can be seen going up into the skull with multiple branches in the brain outlined in the x-ray. On the right side the picture shows brain death. There is contrast in the artery in the neck, stopping at the base of the skull, with no flow upwards into the brain. No blood vessels are seen inside the skull. This is the picture of brain death where brain swelling has choked off blood supply to itself. Persistence of this situation results in brain death. (Picture taken from www.donorrecovery.org. used with permission from FusionSpark Media Inc)

None of the fancy tests had proved superior to the Harvard Criteria which were simple to do, and could be done at little or no cost at the patient's bedside.

Major Deepak, driving to the hospital in the middle of the night, was not concerned with the Upanishads, nor was he interested in what they were saying or doing in Harvard. He wanted to make sure the Indian law was going to be properly followed, and he remembered from a refresher course he had attended in the Army, that Parliament had passed the law governing brain death in 1994. There had been considerable debate regarding it at the time, and legal clarifications had been sought. Henceforth death could be diagnosed in two ways, they had been informed during the refresher course: either by way of cardiac death, or brain death. This was what he wanted to check on his computer as soon as he got to his office.

Dr. Google confirmed everything he had been taught in the fauj. Taking a print-out, he marched to the ICU to meet the doctors assembled and waiting there.

The Night Duty doctor was the most cheerful of the group. The Critical Medicine Specialist and the Neurosurgeon were ignoring each other, the hostility between them, obvious.

"May I ask, what is the need to diagnose brain death in this case, Sir?" the Neurosurgeon asked grumpily, "We have never done this in the past in this hospital. In fourteen years of practicing Neurosurgery, I have never done this testing."

"No testing. Really? Then how am I to know someone is going to recover from coma or is brain dead?" asked Maj. Deepak with a piercing look at the Neurosurgeon

"It is a matter of experience, Sir," the Neurosurgeon said, refusing to meet his stare.

The implication that a Hospital Administrator lacked experience to make a Neurological judgment was not lost on Maj. Deepak. At no time of day, and especially at 2 AM in the morning, was he willing to tolerate insolence.

"Experience. Experience? I am sorry, doctor. From now on, the diagnosis of death in this hospital will be made according to scientific principles, and the statutory requirements will be met. We either do things properly or we don't do them at all." Maj. Deepak had crescendoed into his parade ground voice, and everyone within earshot wilted.

"Do you know, doctors," he continued, handing out copies of the documents he had printed, "It is mandatory, since 2012, in Kerala, to diagnose brain death in exactly the manner it is prescribed in law? Please read it."

He handed out the print-outs he had taken. (see Appendix 3)

"This is exactly what I have been asking for here, Sir," said the Critical Care Medicine Specialist, emboldened by the support he was getting from the Chief.

"OK. You both know what needs to be done. Please proceed," ordered the Major.

When Sunita arrived at the hospital there was an urgent call waiting for her from the ICU. It was the ICU nurse.

"Last night they did the tests on Jose, and he is brain dead!"

"Oh that is terrible! His poor wife! What will she do?"

"That is why I am calling you," continued the nurse, "I want you here when she gets here. I had sent her home last night saying Jose was stable and nothing more was going to be done so there was no point in her staying here in the waiting room. I thought she needed to rest, and I told her to go home. Oh my God, what will she say now?"

"Don't worry. I will talk to her. It may have been a good thing she was not here when this actually happened. What do they plan to do with Jose now?"

"I don't know!" wailed the nurse, "I have never had to deal with such a situation! Oh, why did this have to happen today?"

Although Sunita was maintaining her composure, she too was nonplussed. What was the next thing to do?

She decided that Maj. Deepak was the best person to advise her. She thought it would be better to meet with him before meeting the family members.

Maj. Deepak was in his office. He appeared obviously red eyed and sleep deprived.

"What will we do? We are going to repeat the tests 6 hours after the first set of brain death tests. So that will happen about 9 or 10 AM. After that we will inform the patient's family members."

"And then what happens, Sir?" asked the Social Worker.

"What happens? What happens is what always happens when someone dies in hospital. The family takes the body home."

"But this is a medicolegal case, Sir. The police have to be informed, and there will have to be a post mortem examination by the Police surgeon."

"Medicolegal. Hmm." None of the doctors in the middle of the night had thought about this problem. "Post mortem, yes. All that can be done. Why do you ask?"

Maj. Deepak was thinking on the fly, and was hoping for some answers himself.

"Sir, I was only clarifying. Everyone is a little confused as to what is to be done" was all he got from his Social Worker.

Maj. Deepak knew what to do when there was confusion all around: Attack! This was standard military strategy.

"Confused! Confusion? There will be no further confusion! In such cases, the procedure to be followed is very clear. Proper diagnosis must be done! None of this business of quietly reducing care or withdrawing support based on somebody's impressions about whether the coma is irreversible or not, or can the patient survive or not. Dammit, we are living in the 21st century now! Get used to the proper way of doing things! All confusion will end when you do things properly!"

"Very good, Sir," Sunita retreated hastily from the lair of the enraged bear.

Back in the ICU, Sunita found Jose's nurse quite agitated.

"The wife is here," she said, whispering loudly even though Sunita could see nobody within hearing distance, "and she has brought her daughter as well! I didn't tell them anything! I didn't know what to say!"

Hurrying to the waiting room, Sunita saw Seleena sitting against the far wall, in a shadow. Standing beside her was a young girl about 7 or 8 years old, dressed in her Sunday best with a bright pink ribbon in her hair. Sunita could see Seleena was sobbing with her face in her hands. The little girl was facing her mother and trying to comfort her.

Sunita hurried to their side and sat down on the bench next to Seleena and put her arms around her shaking shoulders, holding her close in a sideways embrace. She was facing the daughter who looked at her with wide innocent eyes, a steady gaze, and a serious expression.

"Hello! I am Sunita Aunty. I met your mother yesterday. You must be her daughter. What's your name?"

"My name is Priya Jose," came the answer with eyebrows lifted and a slight smile turning up the corners of her little lips. She stood straight with her hands by her side, and when she said her name she seemed to stand a little straighter, her slender physique showing pride in who she was. Daddy's girl, thought Sunita to herself.

"Oh, you are so pretty! And so well behaved!"

"Thank you Aunty", came the reply. Priya spoke careful sentences, very correctly, as though she was reciting answers in a classroom.

Seleena had been watching her daughter during the exchange, through wet eyes, her sorrow temporarily eased by pride in her daughter, and the good impression she was making.

"I came to see my Daddy. Mummy said I could miss school today. But I will have to take a leave letter tomorrow for my class teacher."

"Oh dear, yes. I am sure we can organize official leave for you."

"They have covered my Daddy's eyes," said the little girl cupping her little hands over her own eyes to show what she had noticed. "And there is a tube in his nose. And another tube in his mouth."

"Yes, my dear. You noticed everything. What a clever girl!"

Sunita's heart felt like it would burst with the sadness of what she knew, and the news she had come to convey. She turned her attention to the mother.

"How are you, Seleena, did you get any rest last night?"

"No, I couldn't sleep at all. I kept seeing Jose. I don't know if I was dreaming or awake. Then suddenly after about 2 in the morning, there was nothing. That made me even more scared. I wanted to come here right away. But I had to wait till morning. I dropped my son off with his grandparents and came here. But I couldn't bear to come alone, so I brought Priya with me."

"We need to talk. Let's go to my office. We will be more comfortable there and I can make you a cup of coffee."

Sunita was doing more than just being nice to Seleena. She was trying to separate the two from the scene of the tragedy. It would help them to think more clearly about all that she had to tell them. In fact, before she told them anything, she had to understand what was in their minds. She had to make them talk.

"Well," she started carefully, after they had sipped their coffee and approved the sugar was right, "what did you think of Jose when you saw him this morning?"

"Everything looks about the same. The nurse said his BP was a little low around midnight, but they gave him some more fluids, and it came up. But something has changed. I don't know what it is. I can't put my finger on it, but there is a change, and it feels like something serious to me. I thought the nurse is hiding something."

"Yes there is a change, Seleena" sighed Sunita, "his coma got even more deep overnight. His brain is not working. In fact all the senior doctors were here last night and about 4 AM they had to so some tests to figure out what was going on."

"And what did they find?"

"It does not look good."

"Will he recover?"

"At this point they don't think so. But they want to repeat the tests to be sure."

"When will they do that?"

"It will be about 10 o'clock."

"Is he going to live?"

"That is the question they are trying to answer. The tests they did last night suggest that he may not."

"Last night?"

"I mean around 4 AM this morning."

"Yes. Things changed about 2 AM." Seleena sounded convinced of this. "The nurse said his BP dropped about that time. And his urine output which was going so good has slowed down since then."

"You are right. That's about when the change occurred for the worse."

"Will he live? Tell me what you think."

Sunita realized she was being put on the spot. No lying or half truths would work now.

"The tests the senior doctors did last night were to see if his brain is dead. They were positive. The diagnosis now is that he is brain dead."

Seleena eyes were filling up again. She stared intently through her tears at the Social Worker as she reached out to her daughter and hugged her close.

"So he is not going to recover. He is not going to get out of here."

"No."

"Oh God!" Seleena wailed, "he is not going to live. Priya, Daddy is not coming home with us." She clutched her daughter tightly. The little girl had her arms around her mother's head, her eyes wide, taking in the information. She had paid close attention throughout the conversation.

Sunita waited for the sobbing to cease. There was no hurry. Her training had taught her to recognize the different stages of grief, and she knew that an important stage had been reached in the grieving process: acceptance.

Seleena had accepted, albeit with tremendous sorrow and a broken heart, that her husband was dead. Many important things remained to be understood, and life would never be the same again for the mother and daughter in front of her, but for now they just needed some time and space to grieve, and cope with their pain.

Shortly after 10 AM, when the ICU nurse called for Seleena, Sunita and Priya accompanied her to the Conference Room to talk to the Neurosurgeon.

Sunita watched Seleena and Priya carefully as the Neurosurgeon broke the news.

He started off by saying that when Jose had been brought to the hospital he had sustained a very severe injury. His Glasgow Coma Score was less than 8, and that was an indication he had suffered a severe injury to his brain. The CT scan had showed fractures of his skull, and there was an accumulation of blood pressing on his brain. This bleeding had to be stopped and the pressure relieved before they could say anything about the primary injury and how severe it was. The younger the individual, the better his chances of recovery. However, in Jose's case even though he was young, the brain injury had been too severe to survive. Unfortunately, this is often the case in road accidents. The magnitude of the impact is devastating to the human body. Now, he was brain dead. They had suspected it in the night when the ICU nurse had noticed he had stopped responding. They had done the tests to confirm the diagnosis. When the ventilator was stopped he did not breathe. They had waited 10 minutes. Normally nobody can stop breathing for even 1 minute. During the time they waited for him to breathe, his blood gas reports were checked, and showed that the CO_2 level had gone up sufficiently to stimulate breathing. But that had not happened. Loss of the ability to breathe is a vital function of the brain, and without it, there is no life.

Seleena remained very calm throughout the discourse. Most of what she was hearing, she already knew from the updates and explanations given earlier. She had barely heard the Neurosurgical lecture she had just received. She had been more intent on watching the Neurosurgeon than listening. When he had finished, she knew what she needed to know.

It was a hopeless situation, and the doctors could do nothing about it.

The neurosurgeon, having said what he came to say, prepared to leave. Sunita was unwilling to let him go so easily.

"Seleena, this is the time to ask questions," she prompted.

Seleena remained quiet, lost in her thoughts. The Neurosurgeon, sitting down again, was clearly relieved there were no outbursts of crying and wailing.

He has no idea how much work has gone into this, thought Sunita silently to herself.

"Why are my Daddy's eyes covered up?"

The little voice caught everyone by surprise.

"What?" asked the Neurosurgeon, nonplussed at the sudden question shooting from a direction he had left unprotected.

"Why are they covered?" asked little Priya, clearly and more loudly this time.

"Uh, hmm, we always cover the eyes. It's to protect them."

"Can they be used by someone who is blind, to make them see?"

The little girl's question was clear, her small voice like crystal. It burst over the speechless hush of the assembled adults like the detonation of a distant firecracker. The words they had just heard hung over them as though somewhere overhead a Diwali rocket had exploded. And in the stunned silence, a strange illumination, an incandescence like a pyrotechnic shower of fireflowers descending, lighting up the darkness in the room and in everyone's mind.

Seleena was staring with wide eyed astonishment through her welling tears at her daughter. The ICU nurse who had been silent and standing off to one side burst out crying. There was not a dry eye in the room. Even the hardened neurosurgeon had to cough to hide his amazement at the child and how she could look beyond the sad situation, and think of the grief of others who she did not even know.

"Yes, yes. His eyes are fine. In fact all his organs are working fine. Yes. Donation is possible. Of course! If that is what you wish. I think our Social Worker will be able to explain all that." The Neurosurgeon beat a hasty retreat.

PART III

THE OPERATION

Soon after KNOS-Mrithasanjeevani in Trivandrum was informed of the decision to donate all organs made by Jose Avirachen's wife Seleena, there was an explosion of activity in the hospital the like of which had never been witnessed before. This was the first time a multiple organ donation was going to take place here.

There were potential recipients for all the organs. The news spread like wildfire through the corridors, wards, and clinics. Time was of the essence, because after brain death multi-organ failure inevitably follows. If lives were to be saved, Jose's organs had to be retrieved speedily and expeditiously. Everyone knew that, and that was enough to get everyone's adrenaline pumping.

Someone spread a rumor that teams of doctors and nurses from different Transplant centers were on their way and would soon come rushing in. The very prospect was frightening for a hospital accustomed to a sedate pace from 9 AM to 5 PM, check in and check out. Specialist heart surgeons would be coming, someone said! This was unbelievably exciting in a hospital accustomed to seeing a new member of medical staff only once in a bluemoon and then taking a couple of years to get used to him or her.

Some had never seen a cardiac surgeon before. Someone said they never travelled by road, they only flew to wherever they had to go! The hospital engineer heard about it and came rushing in from home to say that the terrace of the hospital would not support a helicopter landing. Don't even think about it! Nursing Supe called for an emergency meeting of all nursing staff. The Labor Room nurses did not think they needed to waste their time attending the meeting, and immediately a discussion started about their insubordination having crossed all limits. Supervisors of different areas put all routine work on hold supposedly to accommodate the transplant. The ENT surgeon stormed into Major Deepak's office demanding to know why his Clinic nurses had disappeared.

"Nurses? What nurses?" said Maj. Deepak warming up a little slowly after his long night of hard work. "Call Nursing Supe and ask her to locate them!"

The ICU and Operation Theater had become a beehive of activity, with some bees in a tearing hurry and others buzzing around in circles. This was all a completely new and at times bewildering experience for everyone. Not everyone has a natural affinity for experiences that are the opposite of old and boring. Nurses in scrub suits drifted around glassy eyed and in a daze, wondering how to set up a cardiac Operation Theater at short notice. In Kerala, however, there is no dearth of people waiting to rush to wherever the action is. When located, the ENT clinic nurses were found waiting outside the ICU, on their marks, crouched and ready to charge in and help should the need arise.

Havildar Nambiar, Maj. Deepak's Trauma Coordinator, called the police to come in and expedite the inquest proceedings. The policeman who wandered in scratched his ears, then his nose, and while examining his finger tip to identify his copious gleanings, announced that he refused to allow the organ donation to proceed. He had never heard of something as irregular as taking organs out of a police case.

Nambiar looked steadily at him for a while thinking to himself how much he would like to break this slovenly cop's neck.

Instead, he called KNOS and was directed to a Director General of Police in Trivandrum, who got on the phone to the Head of Forensic medicine of Trivandrum Medical College to clarify the procedure. The Forensic Prof, a lady doctor who was also a DGP, with a reputation for not mincing her words when dealing with rank and file, gave clear instructions: Not only would the police permit organ donation, but they were ordered to facilitate everything that was needed including the autopsy and early release of the body. The paperwork they needed to complete was something they should know well by this time, and if they did not know it, they could find it in the police manual.

Nambiar took great pleasure inviting the policeman who had baulked back into his office to educate him about his duties. He had been doing some reading of the law in the meantime, and had armed himself with some of the jargon. Legally the police did not get automatic possession of the deceased in a so-called medicolegal case. The body belonged to the next-of-kin. It was of course the democratic duty of those in possession to facilitate inquest proceedings. And they would do so, when asked politely, he said to the hapless policeman before him, swelling his chest and curling his moustache as he delivered the punch line. India is not a police state, he added pungently.

A Neuro specialist from outside the hospital had to be called in to verify the diagnosis of brain death before organ donation could proceed. At first nobody knew there was such a provision in the law. Then nobody knew who to call. A local Neurosurgeon in another hospital said he was willing to come, but he was not on the 'panel' of approved Neurospecialists of the government.

Maj. Deepak got on the phone, now literally a hotline, to KNOS, and was told that they would immediately 'empanel' the Neurosurgeons in his hospital and the neighborhood. The hospital would also be immediately designated a Non Transplant Organ Retrieval Center(NTORC), and the paperwork required for it would be faxed to his office immediately.

KNOS soon submitted to Maj. Deepak the names, designations, and medical licence numbers of the surgeons who would be coming to his hospital for organ retrieval with an official request for temporary privileges. He was asked for permission for a team of cardiac anesthesiologists and Intensivists to come immediately as an advance party to the ICU to work on evaluating the heart and optimizing cardiac function before proceeding to the Operating Theater.

Three teams would be coming: the heart team, the liver team, and the kidney team. There would be 6 surgeons operating simultaneously. Their support staff would include anesthetists, and OT technicians. He would have to organize their largest operating room to accommodate this deluge. Shaking off his grogginess and lack of sleep Maj. Deepak went into overdrive firing orders, organizing teams and facilities, his cell phone constantly ringing, his physical person a mobile command center as he raced around the hospital to make sure everything was optimal.

Sunita stayed with Seleena, Priya and assorted members of the Avirachen family who had showed up, keeping them informed of all that was going on.

There is no helicopter service available in Kerala for transplant teams, but the team of cardiac intensivists got the next best thing: a police escort to lead them, sirens screaming through the glutinous traffic. They turned into the entrance of the hospital with tires squealing. Unloading half a dozen boxes they marched through the foyer and took the stairs two at a time to reach the ICU.

With a quick round of introductions to the ICU nurses and the CCM doctors the Cardiac Intensivists went into action. They pulled monitors and machines out of their bags and positioned them all around Jose's bed. There was a frantic search for extension cords and multi-plug socket boards to facilitate the surge in electricity consumption. Soon Jose had a trans-esophageal echocardiogram probe, a bedside cardiac output monitor, a half dozen new iv and arterial lines, and a Swan Ganz catheter being placed to check the right heart pressure, and do a confirmation of cardiac output and peripheral vascular resistance. His blood pressure medicines were overhauled based on the new information obtained, and fresh infusion pumps started to get the appropriate cardiac drugs on board. Suddenly the heart rate which had been rising came down and the blood pressure stabilized.

The CCM doctor and ICU nurses watched with fascination. Seeing how a dying heart could be revived was a new experience for them, a fantastic learning experience brought to their hospital from out of the blue.

"I need another 2 hours to get everything under control here," the Cardiac anesthetist called back to the cardiac transplant surgeon waiting at the Heart Center to get word on how the donor heart looked, "but I think this heart is going to be good."

The family of the heart recipient who was in the Cardiac ICU on life support and sinking, was informed that he has a heart offer, and they would be going ahead with the transplant. There were tears of joy and muted cheers outside the cardiac ICU at the Heart Center. They had been preparing for a funeral, and suddenly there was a burst of hope!

The phone had rung at the Aliyar Kunju home at 5 in the morning. It was the Transplant Coordinator with the non-Malayalee accent telling them they might have a liver for Kunju.

The phone in the bedroom had been shifted to Ayesha's side so Kunju could get all the rest he needed, and so it was to Ayesha that the Coordinator spoke. She could not remember when she had so loved to hear a strange accent speaking Malayalam.

An immediate scramble ensued. Raza and Shehnaz were informed, Mustafa was called and they were off to the hospital with Mustafa leaning on the horn all the way. Neither Kunju nor Ayesha told him to slow down or to get off the horn. If they had, he probably would not have obeyed.

At the hospital Kunju was checked through admissions straight through to the Transplant ICU where he was divested of his clothes, handed a bottle of pink medicated soap solution and asked to shower, scrubbing till it was all finished, and given a set of sterile disposable hospital clothes to wear thereafter. He would be moved to the Operation Theater after the surgeons had gone to the donor hospital and inspected the liver to make sure it was good to use.

"Why would they not use it? What earthly reason could there be to turn it down?" asked Ayesha breathlessly.

"It may have too much fat on it. Sometimes in accident cases there may be an injury to the liver that was not suspected. And finally they have to make sure the size will be good for Kunju, and also make sure the anatomy is OK."

These were too many specifics for Ayesha. Waiting alone outside the ICU, she just prayed that everything would be good.

A junior doctor from the Hepatology unit came by to examine Kunju, and get his signature on the consent forms. He called Dr. E and gave him the gist of his findings.

Dr. E asked for Kunju to be put on the line.

"Everything looks good for you to go to the Operating Room", he said, "We will be shifting you after the surgeon calls back from the donor hospital."

Kunju thanked the doctor, and lay back in bed in the crinkly and uncomfortable clothes. He was hyperalert, not nervous, and his mind had blanked out his strange surroundings like he used to when they went to a new town for a tournament. He rolled his shoulders and swung his neck from side to side, limbering up as he would before entering the ring. This was going to be the fight of his life. He knew he only needed to focus on what was directly before him.

When the two hour period the cardiac Intensivists had asked for was over, they cleared the donor for surgery.

Seleena and Priya came to the ICU and stood by Jose's bed to say good bye. Priya was holding her mother's hand tightly with both of her own. With her other hand Seleena clutched her husband's hand. It was cold and lifeless, and she wanted to let go, but could not. After some time she felt Sunita tugging at her side, and transferred her grip to the warm proferred hand allowing herself to be comforted and guided out of the ICU.

The Cardiac team that had left the bedside for family goodbyes to be completed came back and took over, disconnecting the ventilator and attaching an Ambu bag to ventilate manually while wheeling the body to the Operating Room. A small platoon of nurses surrounded the bed as it rolled, propping up the monitors resting on his bed during transit, pushing IV poles, banked with infusion pumps in layers, moving in slow procession alongside the bed. Like a giant ship casting anchor and moving out of the harbor surrounded by little tug boats, the ICU bed navigated the straits to the Operation Theater.

The muted sounds and solemnity of the last moments in the ICU, and during transfer, disappeared inside the Operating Room. There was much to be done and everyone was waiting to start.

Anesthetists gathered up the dozens of lines, identifying them to each other and moving them to the head of the bed before transferring Jose's body to the operating table.

Surgical teams had arrived a few minutes earlier and gone straight to the Operation Theater and were scrubbing in the adjacent area to the room where the organ retrieval would be conducted. The Technicians who would assist them had already scrubbed in, and were busy arranging instruments on sterile tables that were arranged all around the periphery against the wall. There were separate tables and separate scrub techs for the cardiac team and the abdominal surgeons.

At the operating table the 'prep and drape' process was begun. An electric razor whined as hair in the line of incision was clipped from chin to pelvis. Medicated soap was slathered on and scrubbed off leaving the skin from neck to thighs glistening clean and dry. Then a layer of brown antiseptic solution was painted on and sterile drapes applied to exclude everything other than the area of incision. The anesthetists at the head end of the table were screened off, though they could look over to check the progress of the operation and communicate with the surgeons. Ready to start simultaneously, the cardiac and liver surgeons positioned themselves around the table. Primary surgeons on the right side of the body, and on the left, their assistants. At the foot end of the table the scrub nurses and technicians had pulled the tables earlier set against the wall closer to the operating table now surrounded by gleaming instruments.

At a signal from the anesthetists, the operation was begun.

Smoke rose from the skin being opened by electrocautery. Unlike usual operations, no scalpels were used. When so many people are operating at the same time, and nobody is familiar with the operating style of the others, safety is paramount. Knife and and needle-stick injuries to operating personnel, always a concern, are more likely in high stress situations when people unfamiliar with each other are operating together.

There is no concern about skin edges being singed by the electric burn. There would be no need for this incision to heal when the operation was done.

The first task, to inspect the entire body and make sure there is no unsuspected infection or tumor or any other disease that can be transmitted to the recipients of the organs was soon completed. The next task, to inspect each individual organ and make sure it is healthy and suitable for its intended recipient proceeded more slowly, requiring careful dissection to define the anatomy unique to every individual and to look for anomalies that might make the transplant difficult or even hazardous.

Everyone in the room was conscious of the fact that the organ retrieval operation is a complex procedure being conducted on a dead individual who is highly unstable, with a physiological situation completely different from the usual. No organs can be removed that do not already have identified recipients, and everyone in the operating room was conscious of the fact that these recipients are waiting in their respective transplant centers desperate for the news that the donor surgeon has called saying the organ is good to go. A mistake by anyone in the room, and the donor could crash, damaging the organs and potentially even rendering them untransplantable.

The pace would be sedate and calm. Excitement in the Operating Room is never a good thing.

But any drop in blood pressure, any irregularity of the heart rhythm would trigger a swift change in pace. It would become necessary in the shortest time possible, to rapidly cool the body down and remove organs speedily. Surgeons performing a retrieval operation had to be able to operate in unfamiliar surroundings, small hospitals, with inexperienced staff, and still be able to move fast to complete the operation when the situation demanded it.

Before leaving for the hospital where Jose Avirachen lay, the liver transplant surgeon had been told that KNOS had allocated the liver to Mohammed Aliyar Kunju. He had gone over the details available in Mohammed Aliyar Kunju's chart, to make an estimate of the size of the liver he needed based on his height, weight and BMI. He had studied the CT scans to see the anatomy of his blood vessels, and if there were any blocked vessels. This would enable him to properly match the donor and recipient. Size mismatches could make the transplant operation hazardous and even a failure.

Size, usually but not always, could be a predictor of function. Bigger was not better when it came to liver. Fatty liver disease was increasingly being found in the normal population. These livers were large and looked OK, but wash out the blood and they would look a sickly yellow. The donor surgeon would have to make a judgment of how the liver would work by looking at its size, color, shape and consistency – all of which were important in making a visual assessment about the approximate degree of fatty change that was present in the liver – not an easy or even accurate exercise. It took years of experience to make a good judgment. Doing a biopsy is one way of bringing objectivity to the life-and-death decision, but this is not easy to do when the donor is located in a peripheral hospital. Biopsies, especially the rapid ones, called 'frozen section' biopsy, are difficult to interpret and notoriously misleading when assessing a liver.

In the case of donor Jose Avirachen, the 'Chief', who the Aliyar Kunju family called 'Dr. A', had decided to waive the liver biopsy prior to accepting the liver. Jose was young, he was not overweight, had little to no alcohol consumption, and his liver blood tests were normal.

"Call me when you see the liver", were his instructions from home to the donor surgeon before he left. And when he heard the report from the donor hospital that it looked good, he called the Operation Theater at the Transplant center. The nurse who picked up the phone had already been alerted about the possibility that there would be a liver transplant that day. She had been informed that the recipient was admitted and waiting in the

ICU. When the phone rang and she recognized the voice of Dr. A on the line, she could almost anticipate the order that came,

"Send for the patient!".

At the donor hospital, a crucial stage of the operation had been reached: they were ready for cross-clamp.

The sound of hammering as ice was broken filled the Operating Room. The ice was really frozen iv saline contained in special double layer bags. Not every hospital has an ice making machine to make sterile ice-slush. Orthopedic mallets were used to pound on the bags and break the sterile (salty) ice into small pieces to pack into the body and surround the organs to help cool them down.

Until better ways are found to preserve organs, the principle is to keep them cool, slow down the multiple cellular processes that constitute the term 'metabolism', and hope they will recover when the organ is warmed up again in the recipient. The process of cooling the organ is accomplished by first cannulating (inserting large bore tubes into) the aorta and infusing cold solutions that will wash out the blood. This cools all organs at their core. The ice packed around each organ cools the surface.

The cardiac and liver surgeons had struck up a good partnership in the course of Jose Avirachen's multi-organ retrieval. The liver is located in the upper abdomen close to the heart, and the largest vein in the body, the inferior vena cava(IVC) that returns blood from the lower body to the right side of the heart runs behind and almost through the liver to reach the heart. The distance between the liver and the heart is negligible, and in retrieving one, it is easy to damage the other. Ugly scenes have resulted with hypercompetitive surgeons trying to upstage one another. In this case, however the two were cordial and agreed on the site at which the cardiac surgeon would divide the large vein so that each surgeon would have enough to hook up in his recipient.

A cardiac transplant is actually one of the easiest operations for a skilled cardiac surgeon. Repairing a heart is usually much more difficult than replacing it entire. It is possible to work with a very short length of the IVC or even none at all, but cardiac surgeons like to keep this a closely guarded secret, and the length of the IVC is often the bone for the big dog to snarl over and intimidate the smaller dog.

In this case the cardiac surgeon was in a generous mood.

"Is that much vein enough for you?" he asked.

"Yes it is, thank you," said the liver surgeon, happily.

"Any more, and I will be giving you a bit of the heart as well," answered the cardiac guy, unable to resist a little dig, "your liver might start beating and making funny sounds, dub-dub, lub-dub."

"Oh, we will just say we've done a combined heart-liver transplant," answered the liver surgeon, not to be outdone at being smart-alecky, "we can always add a little extra to the bill."

The mood was light. A good place to be before the most tense part of the operation.

"Ready for heparin" the cardiac surgeon said to the anesthetist.

"Thirty thousand?

"Yes".

Thirty thousand units of heparin is an industrial dose. The usual dose is a maximum of about 5000 units for an average size person. But this was a dead person, and the only side effect – bleeding – was not a concern. What was important was to make sure no blood clotted and destroyed the micro-circulation within the organs. The fine skein of vessels dispersed throughout the body, coursing through every layer and structure, and ultimately getting through to each and every cell, has been estimated to have a total length of 60,000 miles, or 100,000 kms. That's a lot of territory for clot to form. That's a lot of heparin needed.

Three minutes after the heparin was in, the aorta, the largest blood vessel coming out of the heart, was clamped, and perfusion with cold solution was begun via the cannulae (tubes) earlier placed within the aorta. Core cooling had begun.

The theater erupted into a cacophony of loud voices. Technicians monitoring the rate at which preservative solution was flowing into the organs began calling out to the surgeons telling them whether the fluid was flowing well or not. The amount that had flowed in was also called out periodically.

"Cardioplegia flowing well!" to the cardiac surgeon.

"Aorta not flowing good! Portal vein flowing well," to the liver surgeon.

"How's it going now?" after the liver surgeon made some adjustments.

"Better….. Little better….. OK! Now going good!"

"How much is in?" asked the liver surgeon

"Two liters aortic, one liter portal!"

"Give me more ice. I want more ice!"

"More ice coming up!"

"Break some more ice!"

"Liver looks good, perfusing well. It has a good color!"

"More ice around the heart!"

The heart was looking good to the cardiac surgeon. It looked awful to everybody else. A heart that has stopped beating is not something one sees every day in the operating room. As the cardioplegia solution flowed in, the electrolyte concentrations it contained caused the heart muscle to relax and then to stop beating altogether.

Blood flowing out of the organs poured from the IVC into the chest, and was evacuated by large bore suction tubes. The noise of three suckers going full blast added to the general cacophony in the room.

"Hold it! This suction bottle is full!"

"Change the bottle! Hurry up! I need suction!"

The noise of suckers is always an ominous sound during an operation, as it usually indicates bleeding and the surgeon needs the blood sucked out of the field in order to be able to see the bleeding vessel and control it. In this situation it was a happy sound. It was the sound of an organ retrieval operation continuing successfully to its most important stage. Blood was being replaced by preservation solution. Organs were being cooled down at their core by cold fluid, and on the surface by ice chips packed into the body and surrounding each individual organ that would be retrieved. It was the sound which signals the beginning of the final stage of the operation: to remove the organs that would save lives.

Noting the time the aorta was cross-clamped and the cold perfusion started, sets the clock for every transplant. From now on, for each transplant team, the time on the clock and whether it was day or night, or a Tuesday in January, was of no consequence. The only thing that mattered now was the "cold ischemia time": the time before the organs would be reperfused with blood in the recipient's body, reestablishing the conditions necessary for them to resume normal function.

Every effort would be made to keep the cold ischemia time as short as possible.

Removing the organs as quickly as possible and packaging them was the first step.

The heart was the first to be removed. With a large scissors the cardiac surgeon cut through the vessels running into and out of each side of the heart, and lifted it out of the chest. There was a scramble to get a basin with sterile bags packed in ice chips and slush to pack the heart. Three layers of sterile high quality imported plastic bags (each costing nearly a thousand rupees) would be used around the heart. Called "triple bagging", this would maintain sterility during transit.

The cardiac surgeon shook gloved hands with the liver surgeon who still had work to do, in a small farewell ceremony that is customary for transplant teams before leaving the OR.

"Good luck with your patient" he said to the liver surgeon.

"Good luck to you too," came the reply before the liver surgeon returned his entire attention to his task of dissecting the donor liver's blood vessels before taking it out, "and travel safe!"

Traveling safe is always of paramount concern to transplant surgeons. Though rare, crashes have regularly occurred worldwide, resulting in the death of transplant teams and loss of the organs they were transporting. Rushing to get the organ to the recipient can make for careless driving.

In the Heart Hospital where the recipient was located, the cardiac surgeon performing the recipient operation had already started work. Putting the patient on cardiopulmonary bypass and taking out his diseased heart to make way for the new one, could be a time consuming procedure. Coordinating the two operations was key to keeping the cold ischemia time of the heart low. The goal was to get the heart beating again within six hours, preferably within four. That is not a long period of time, and not more than an hour can be spent travelling. Cardiac transplant surgeons need helicopters and Lear jets if the distances they have to cover are long or if the roads are slow.

"Time flies when you are having fun" was the aphorism for transplant surgeons. It was dictum and warning, not a happy observation. They could not afford to get carried away with what they were doing. They had to keep watching the clock, get things done and keep moving.

"The enemy of good is perfect", was another aphorism drilled into a trainee transplant surgeon. You can always find a better way of doing something, and get it to look better, or more perfect. But if it was going to take more time, it was probably not worth it.

In Kerala, no plans for air transport of transplant teams have been made. Helicopters, status symbols for rich businessmen dabbling in jewelry, wedding garments, and hotels stand idle in airport parking spots and hangars. Even if they were made available, the Navy would probably object. Objecting to civilian aircraft flying into their protected air space was what the Navy and Air force routinely did. It saved them trouble. Consistently successful in grounding the persons who paid the taxes to make their very existence possible, the uniformed forces in India had made it too complicated for anyone to even think of organizing air transport for transplantation.

Fortunately, Kerala state police have stepped into the breach, and cooperate to make charging through crowded roads as safe as possible. A police escort was waiting for the cardiac team as they hurried out of the hospital entrance with their icebox containing the heart, and the boxes of equipment they had brought with them and now had to take back.

With the police car in the lead, overhead light flashing, and the ambulance with the cardiac team following, the convoy moved out of the hospital compound. As they hit the road the sirens came on parting traffic and deafening everybody as they accelerated down the road.

In the donor hospital OR, the liver surgeon was close to getting done. Cutting out the liver (the official term is 'explant') is not as easy as the heart, and for this part of the operation he donned his operating telescopes and a headlight to be able to better see the delicate structures he had to locate and preserve. Notorious for variations in anatomy, blood vessels to the liver can be single or multiple, and the surgeon has to spot these and avoid mishaps. It is the most trying part of the procedure, and with the blood washed out, nothing looks familiar. Arteries to the liver are 'end-arteries' and if damaged, parts of the liver, or even the entire organ can die, with life threatening consequences for the recipient. Need for retransplantation, or even death can result from a minor or unnoticed error during organ retrieval.

After the liver was removed from Jose's body, it was examined again on a table off to the side of the operating room. It was called, naturally, the 'backtable'. Backtabling the liver would be done twice: Once here in the donor hospital and again after reaching the recipient transplant center. Here the most important task was to perfuse another liter of perfusion fluid into the main vein that enters the liver – called the portal vein, and wash out the last traces of blood contained in the liver and replace it all with the preservation fluid called UW solution.

UW (for University of Wisconsin) solution is a concoction first developed in the early 1980s, and popularized worldwide by the end of the decade. UW solution has remained "state of the art" for well over thirty years. It has also held its price. Introduced at $200 per liter, it was sold now at $250 per liter even after the patent has run out. Alternatives and generic equivalents have not been popular with liver surgeons who refused to compromise on cost if it put their patient's life at risk. The cost of the perfusion of all the organs in the donor, and then the extra 1 L on the backtable for the portal vein would run to a few hundred thousand rupees per donor.

No mechanism has been worked out to pay for all the materials and manpower hours spent on each donor. Kerala, like the rest of India is still trapped in a socialist mindset when it comes to health care and medical services. The government is supposed to provide it free of cost. In reality, government hospitals in India provide mostly substandard care at enormous cost to the taxpayer.

Two government medical college hospitals in Kerala were doing kidney transplants, and every time there was a donor in a private hospital one kidney was mandatorily allocated to a patient in a government medical college transplant center. Ironically, Kerala government hospitals and medical colleges almost never motivate organ donation. This was not for lack of potential organ donors as there was always a steady stream of head injury patients admitted via their Casualty Departments. They rarely did what was necessary to look after a catastrophic neurological injury patient well enough to lead to organ donation. Even in Trivandrum Medical College, where KNOS was started, Neurosurgeons would refuse, on a daily basis, to certify brain death preferring to let 'nature take its course' and allow precious organs to fail slowly.

Institutes of national importance like Sri Chitra in Kerala, and NIMHANS in Bangalore (the National Institute of Mental health and Neurosciences), maintained at enormous expense to the taxpayer, are supposed to set the standards in Neurosciences for the rest of the country. Here too the familiar pattern is seen. The prevalent practice is refusal to participate in organ donation. In the twenty years since the Human Organ Transplant Act has been passed, not a single organ donation has taken place in NIMHANS.

All over India, potential organ donors with catastrophic brain injury, on a daily basis, are made to lie in a corner untended or minimally tended till all organs fail and the heart arrests. At which time they are parceled off to nearby Forensic Medicine departments for medico-legal autopsy and disposal.

The scientific community in India, numerically the largest in the world, famous for self sufficiency in its space program, and high tech capability in warfare including the research, development, and indigenous production of the fastest supersonic cruise missile in the world, appears to have gone adrift in the medical field where waste, corruption, inefficiency and complacency about lack of progress is the norm.

In a democratic country developing nuclear weapons, cruise missiles, satellites and space rockets; where, in fact, rocket science was reality, and a rocket scientist had even been President; where people live who regularly figure at the top of lists of the richest people in the world, and salaried middle class tax-payers are numerically greater than the entire population of many advanced countries, the glib excuse for organization of medical care that is mired in the middle ages is: "no money". Advanced medical care was not for common folk. The few that need expensive treatments like transplant could find the money for it, and look after themselves.

When the Kidney retrieval surgeons had finished removing the kidneys *en bloc* from Jose Avirachen's body, they too worked on their backtable to separate the kidneys. They chose one for their patient, packaging the other to be transported to the government hospital to which KNOS mandatorily allocates one kidney.

The last step of the retrieval procedure was for the liver surgeons to do. They came back to remove the iliac vessels: blood vessels that ran down from the abdomen to the legs. They could use them in their recipient should the blood vessels to the liver be diseased or otherwise unsuitable.

With all their treasures neatly 'triple bagged', and packed in ice in insulated boxes, the surgeons who had completed the organ retrieval left the hospital to hit the road and head back to their respective transplant centers in the shortest time possible.

The last organs to be retrieved in the donation process, were actually the first that the family had wanted to donate: his eyes.

The eye retrieval team had come from the Eye Bank located in Angamali, and worked quietly after the anesthetists had relinquished their place at the head of the operating table. They retrieved the corneas, and meticulously sutured the eyelids closed. The bruising remained, but the swelling seemed to have decreased around his eyes, considerably improving his appearance. His head bandages covering the incision made by Neurosurgeons were replaced fresh and now looked like a white skull cap.

Jose Avirachen's body, washed and dressed, was ready to be handed over to his relatives. Brought back to the ICU where he was admitted prior to going to the OT, he looked a little pale, but was otherwise unchanged. He was dressed in the clothes Seleena had brought: his favorite white shirt and cream colored mundu. Together with his (new) white headgear, his last appearance that Seleena would always carry in her mind, was that of a pilgrim heading out for some holy shrine.

The ICU nurses, extremely apprehensive throughout this new experience of organ donation, and in a tizzy since the moment they had left their patient in the Operating Room, were visibly relieved when they saw the body after donation. The experience had not been as traumatic as anticipated, and had actually been quite good. They recalled many occasions when they had a similar patient and had drifted along day after day not knowing where they were headed, certain of a poor outcome when surgical intervention had failed to improve the patient's neurological status, feeling guilty at having to keep up appearances or make false promises to relatives left in limbo. His wife standing by his side looked calm and dry eyed. Like them, she too seemed happy with the way everything had gone. There was a calm in the ICU, a feeling of closure for everyone who had worked on Jose Avirachen at the end of his life.

One thing however had not changed for the ICU nurses: they had to make sure the bills were paid before they could release the body to the relatives. Nursing Supe had already called them to make sure they knew they were not to release the body until every last penny had been paid. Accordingly she had informed the Accounts section and the final bill had been hand delivered to the ICU. An eye popping amount was still owed to the hospital. Hesitatingly, the nurses handed Seleena her hospital bill.

When she saw the bill, Seleena felt faint and had to sit down quickly. There was a choking sensation in her throat, as though someone had reached from behind and was strangling her. She would have to sell their house if she was going to ever pay up the amount owed. What was going to happen to her and the children?

The ICU nurses, trained to recognize shock, were alarmed at the abrupt deterioration in Seleena's appearance, and her obvious dizzy spell, after she saw the bill. Someone had a bright idea and called Sunita. This was a job for the Social Worker, surely.

Unaware of what was going on, Sunita was in her office, speaking on the phone to Hav. Nambiar, familiarizing herself with the medico-legal procedures necessary before the police would get done with their inquest. She wanted to accompany Seleena as she went through the medicolegal ordeal, but was not feeling too confident. Police, and police stations, frightened her. When her cell phone buzzed, she excused herself and told Nambiar she would call him back. What she heard made her go red, and flames to shoot forth from her eyes and ears. Soon she was hurrying out of her office in a rush to get to the ICU and start damage control.

Quickly relieving Seleena of the bill, and telling her not to worry, she would do what she could about it, Sunita marched off to meet Maj. Deepak.

He had had a nap and was looking refreshed. His secretary had ordered him a cup of strong coffee, and sipping it, he leaned far back in his reclining chair gazing out of his picture window at the scene outside. The grass was green, the sky was pleasantly cloudy, and the odd cow grazed, content with its eternal ruminations. Last night did not turn out too badly after all, Maj. Deepak was thinking. He had lost some sleep, but felt none the worse for it. He should probably do this more often. One of the cows turned and looking towards him interrupted her chewing to let out a long moo, wholeheartedly approving this idea.

Behind him, suddenly interrupting his bucolic meditations, there was a commotion. And into arcadia charged his Social Worker, clucking with the ferocity of a mad mother hen.

"Sir, have you seen this bill?"

"Bill. Ah bill. You mean bill? Yes. What bill?" answered the Major, characteristically.

Transplant Story

"The bill, Sir, that Accounts has drawn up for Jose Avirachen!" Sunita was having difficulty being patient. She thrust out the sheaf of lengthy computer printed sheets that she had been flapping as she marched into the office.

"Accounts. Yes. The Accounts Department, you mean! They have been pretty good with bills. I've had no complaints about them. No issues so far."

Clearly, Accounts had the sleep deprived Maj. Deepak's vote of confidence. Sunita decided to change her line of attack.

"Sir, I am not saying there is anything wrong with the bill. Or with the Accounts section. But we have to show some sensitivity in the way we present the bill to the patient."

"Sensitivity. Absolutely. 'Sensitivity makes sense', I always say."

"These nurses, Sir, have no sensitivity. They gave this bill to the wife of the organ donor, and said this has to be paid before they will release his dead body! Can you imagine what that poor woman may be feeling?"

"Yes. Yes. Now I understand what you are getting at. We have to treat sensitive matters with sensitivity. We must have classes in sensitivity for our nurses. Sensitivity Training. Why don't you take up this matter, Sunita? Someone has to take up this matter, and I think you are the best person for the job!"

Sunita cursed silently. She had landed herself with one more responsibility. More work, with no remuneration of course. Meanwhile she had got nowhere on the matter of the unpaid bill for Jose Avirachen which is what she had come for. Maj. Deepak was unlikely to be of much help with this bill. It seemed like a hopeless situation. She would have to find a philanthropic donor to help with these expenses. That was impossible at such short notice. She prepared to ask Maj. Deepak for an order for payment to be deferred, while she tried to raise the money.

Just then the phone rang.

Sunita decided to do Maj. Deepak a favor, though he clearly did not deserve it, and picked up the phone.

"Hello? Administration," she said in her 'official' voice, a couple octaves lower than what she usually pitched when dealing with people in the Administration building.

The caller identified himself.

"Sir, it's a Transplant coordinator. He is calling from the Transplant center," Sunita whispered to Maj. Deepak, covering the mouthpiece with her hand.

Maj. Deepak, unwilling to take the call, did his characteristic verbal procrastination in sign language. Hold on, he signaled, *(pumping the air in front of him with both palms upheld)*. I, pointing to himself, don't want to talk to him, *(index finger on his lips)*. What does he want? *(accompanying hand gesture internationally recognized as 'what the ****?')*

Sunita listened to the voice with the strange Malayalam accent, watching Maj. Deepak's pantomime with idle interest. What she was hearing had grabbed her complete and undivided attention.

Maj. Deepak watched the conversation keenly. Sunita glanced at him now and then, smiling and popping her eyebrows, doing her own little pantomime, as though to tell him – you're not going to believe this!

When the conversation ended, Sunita was smiling.

"That was the Transplant Coordinator from the Transplant Center that is getting the liver," she announced, "Such a sweet chap. Speaks Malayalam with a weird accent though. Wonder where he is from."

Maj. Deepak wished she would get on with it. He could not have cared if the Coordinator's Malayalam accent was from Mars.

"It seems KNOS allows for payment from recipient hospitals to the donor hospital to cover expenses. We will get Rs 1.5 Lakhs right away. Guaranteed."

"Wow! KNOS, wow!" Maj. Deepak could scarcely believe his ears! "That should cover Jose Avirachen's bill!"

"What planet are you living on, Sir? That will not even cover half of the bill! Not to mention the 50,000 bucks his wife has already paid by hocking her jewelry at the pawn shop!"

"Jewelry. Pawned her jewelry? Really? Not a good idea. She will never get it back."

"Oh yes she will. The Coordinator has promised to send me the email IDs and phone numbers of the coordinators at the other hospitals to which organs were allocated. It should be possible to get them all to contribute, and cover the entire bill, including the deposit at the pawn shop. You will have to call Accounts and ask them to refund that fifty thousand rupees, Sir. You can tell them that it is your executive decision. Yes, you can! Meanwhile, I will start making some calls!"

Sunita bustled out of Administration, much happier, but only marginally less aggressive than when she had entered it a short while earlier.

At the Transplant Center, it was about an hour since Kunju had been taken into the Operation Theater. Ayesha had watched him go reluctantly, clutching his hand till the last moment, too choked with emotion to say anything. She had returned to the room that had been allotted to them, and checked out the bathroom and the sheets and towels as she always did in hotels. This is where she would have to be for the next few weeks. Shehnaz and Raza had not been able to get to the hospital in time to see their Dad before he was taken to the OT. It made her feel bad that they had not been able to say goodbye to him. When she realized how negative that thought was, she scolded herself. She wished she had someone to talk to. She decided she needed a coffee. At least the cafeteria was a familiar place where she had been many times with Kunju. She hesitated to go there alone, but decided it would feel better to sit there than in this room all alone.

At the cafeteria, she was surprised to see Krishnan.

They stared at each other across the room, surprised, wondering what the other was doing there at this odd hour. Krishnan came rushing over. He had immediately realized the reason.

"Is it what I think it is? They have a liver for Kunju?"

"Yes!" said Ayesha her melancholy immediately lifted. She was so glad she had decided to come to the cafeteria.

"You must come over to our table. My wife is there," he pointed, "I will get your coffee for you."

At the table, Ayesha was introduced to Mrs. Krishnan. She seemed to be a very formal person, the opposite of Krish. Ayesha was glad Mrs. Krishnan was present. She wanted to talk to Krish, and was sure Kunju would not mind, but she did not want to be seen alone with him in the cafeteria.

"Wow, you must be thrilled!" gushed Krish, his voice so loud, Ayesha was embarrassed someone would overhear and wonder what was going on.

Normally nobody is 'thrilled' in a hospital.

"And you? What are you here for?"

"And that is what is so crazy, I can hardly believe it! I am here for a transplant as well!"

Ayesha stared at him questioningly. What was he saying? Then her eyes widened as realization dawned.

Krish was nodding at her with a huge smile.

"We may have the same donor!"

Ayesha's hands flew to her face, as her jaw literally dropped!

As always, Krish was the one to explain things. He would have to wait for the kidney to arrive and for the results of the 'matching' before he could be sure he was getting the kidney.

He had already gone to the lab and given his blood. They had collected ten tubes once again! Now they would have to wait for the kidney to get here. The donor surgeon removes lymph nodes from the donor, and these are used to get the lymphocytes with which the matching procedure would be done.

Donor cells, and Krishnan's serum would be mixed, and incubated to see if he had antibodies against the donor. Only if he did not, would he get the kidney.

"Then why did they take Kunju into the OT so early? Don't they have to wait to do the matching for him as well?" Ayesha, still unhappy they had taken Kunju to the OT so quickly, was now alarmed. Had they made some mistake?

Krish immediately reassured her. He had been doing some reading about liver transplants in case he needed one in future because of his hepatitis C infection.

"That's the beauty of it!" he told Ayesha, "they don't need to do any matching for the liver! The liver does not get rejected by the immune system the way other organs do. As long as the blood group is OK and the size is right, they can proceed!"

Ayesha was relieved. Trust her not to have known such details. It was all very complicated, and she was so dumb, she scolded herself. Raza and Shehnaz would probably have known though, and would have explained everything, she comforted herself.

"How long before you know the results of your matching tests?" asked Ayesha

"Takes up to 4 hours for the basic testing. Sometimes the initial results are not clear, and they have to run more complex tests, and it can take longer. No hurry for me. I just have to wait."

Krish was suddenly distracted. The table he had chosen was next to a window that overlooked the hospital entrance.

"Here they come!" he said excitedly.

They all looked to where he was pointing. A police car was entering with overhead lights flashing. The siren screamed one last time as the car slowed at the entrance.

Behind it came an ambulance. Doors flew open, and figures clad in hospital scrub suits jumped out. Large ice boxes were hauled out. Someone had run to the entrance and commandeered a patient trolley which was rattling out to the ambulance. Boxes were loaded onto the trolley, and with one person pushing and the others holding on to the boxes protectively to keep them from falling off, the whole troop disappeared into the hospital.

"And there they go!" enthused Krish, still excited, but now with a satisfied tone to his voice.

Ayesha drew a deep breath. There was a constricting sensation in her chest. She had unknowingly been holding her breath while watching the drama unfold downstairs. She wished her children had been with her to witness this. She would never be able to adequately describe it in words to them.

Back at the donor hospital, the day was coming to its scheduled end. It had been an unusual day, a first experience. Maj. Deepak called for a meeting of all the principle participants in the multi-organ donation for a quick debrief before they all left for the day.

First one into the Conference Room in Administration was Nursing Supe. Arriving before all the others, she took a position toward the back of the room where she could hide if she wanted and be seen only if she wanted. Many people had rushed to her during the day to find out what was going on, and she had feigned great disinterest, and ordered them to go about their work as usual. She would rather not have come at all to this meeting, but the Nursing Superintendent was going to be there, she knew, and so she could not be absent. She glanced at her watch hoping this would not take too long. It was already past the time for her to have left for the day.

The Billing and Accounts officer came in, toting a small file. Three ICU nurses followed, in their blue scrub suits. They had never been in this conference room before, and did not know what a 'debrief' was. The boldest one among them led the way and quickly selected the seats where they would sit in a huddle.

Soon the doctors started arriving. The Neurosurgeon, the Critical Care doctor, and two of the Casualty Medical Officers trooped in one by one. The Chief of Anesthesia arrived along with the Nursing Superintendent. The nurses and Nursing Supe stood up and wished them good evening as they entered.

Maj. Deepak, waiting in his office, ever conscious of protocol, was the last one to come in. He had a stranger with him. Everyone assembled in the room rose when he entered.

Asking them all to be seated, he started off without preamble.

"Ladies and Gentlemen, I have called this meeting so that while the day's incidents are fresh in everyone's mind we can discuss the case of Jose Avirachen. Two more individuals are to attend, Medico Social Worker and Trauma Coordinator Nambiar. I have just got a call to tell me they are on the way.

"This is the first time we have diagnosed brain death in this hospital, and I wanted everyone to be clear about the procedure involved. First of all let me introduce to you the person I have here, who many of you may not know. This is the hospital lawyer, Mr. Namboodri. He will start the proceedings with explaining the legal position as regards brain death. Next, I have asked our Chief of Anesthesia and Critical Care Medicine to review the chart of the deceased patient, and go over what happened in the form of a peer review, so that she can analyze what went right and what did not go right or can be improved in future. I want this to be an interactive session, and people should speak up and clarify their doubts.

"The objective of this meeting is for all to understand the legal and medical aspects of this case, and also to review the documentation, so that in future if we encounter a similar case there will be no confusion. Since this patient was also a medicolegal case, it offers a good opportunity for all of us to understand the new legal environment in which we are working. The rules of the game have changed, gentlemen," he said with unction, momentarily forgetting he was also addressing ladies, "and we have to learn to play by them!"

The Lawyer stood up, happy to have the floor, and extracting a sheaf of papers from his briefcase, began a discourse on the law. Maj. Deepak knew he could go on and on for an hour, and glanced at his watch. He would interrupt him in 3 minutes.

At the end of the 3 minutes, the lawyer had just barely hit his stride when Maj. Deepak interrupted, "I think we will start the discussion. Doctor, would you like to start?" he pointed to the Neurosurgeon, and leaned back to enjoy the fun.

Half an hour later, the discussion was continuing animatedly. The Neurosurgeon was clarifying points in the law which he thought the lawyer was confused about. There were many things he found disagreeable about organ transplant legislation, and while he too, like Nursing Supe, had come to this meeting reluctantly, he was glad to have the opportunity and audience to voice in public the things he had hitherto grumbled about privately.

The lawyer on his part, was delighted he had found someone who thought he knew the law but actually did not. This was the kind of situation that could generate business for him.

The Chief of Anesthesia had many points in the chart that, in her opinion, could have been written better. She stressed the point that if something was not documented it meant, for practical purposes that it was not done.

Uniformed cafeteria personnel entered, and served coffee and samosas. Nursing Supe who was getting increasingly impatient as everyone droned on, and was wondering how she could somehow find an excuse to leave, now settled down in her seat more comfortably. She wished the coffee had more sugar, and when Nursing Superintendent was looking the other way, helped herself to another samosa.

"That's her third samosa," whispered one ICU nurse to the others. They had difficulty controlling their giggles.

Suddenly the door opened, the late comers walked in, and the room fell silent.

All eyes turned to Sunita, who was beaming from ear to ear. Never one to keep silent or observe the formalities of a doctor-nurse hierarchy, because she did not belong to either category, she was now bursting with news she could hardly contain.

"I just got a call from the coordinator at the Heart center. Our patient's heart is beating again!"

A cheer broke out in the room. The ICU nurses clapped with excitement.

"And you know what?" Sunita was not done, "he said the heart was working so well, their patient is already off the three drugs he had been needing to keep his blood pressure up. His heart failure has corrected almost immediately!"

The decibel level in the room increased. Sunita, ever the feminist, was going to make sure credit was given where it was due.

"Three cheers for our nurses!"

She went over to hug them.

"The coordinator at the heart center said the cardiac surgeon especially said to say a big Thank you to the ICU staff for the excellent care they took of their patient!"

Everyone applauded the nurses. Only the Neurosurgeon was quiet, looking sullen. Looking, as they famously say in Malayalam, like a squirrel who has lost his nuts.

"How did everything go at the Police Station?" Maj. Deepak asked.

"No-issues, Sir," boomed Hav. Nambiar, "some minor questions about the surgeons' report which they wanted two more copies. We submitted all the original documents to them, with copies in triplicate, and we have also retained copies for our records."

"The Police Surgeon. How was he? Happy?"

"No, not very happy with having to stay late Sir. In the end he did not even have to do the autopsy. Just a quick open and close and of course they had to examine the brain. Completely destroyed, Sir. He said the brain was almost like water pouring out when they opened the skull!"

An audible gasp went around the room.

"And the family members?" prompted Maj. Deepak.

"Oh, they were very happy, Sir. Very happy, because we were there to help them get the post mortem done. No need to bribe anyone. No-issues at all," Nambiar repeated. He loved dealing with 'issues'. Mostly with the intention of smashing them to smithereens, and making them 'no-issues'.

"Ms Sunita and I accompanied the body to the house," Nambiar continued, "wonderful people, Sir, wonderful. The wife, Sir! Hats off to her! Brave!

Bahadur hai, Saab" he added, lapsing into parade ground Hindustani with his senior officer.

"We placed a wreath on the body at their house, Sir," added Sunita, "I had the florist write it was from our hospital. The wife was very appreciative. And, Yes, I agree with Hav. Nambiar, she really deserves a bravery award. We were discussing it. The government should give some special recognition to such families. What is it with all these freedom fighter awards still being handed out? Decades after the British have left India! The widow of this patient should get a freedom fighter award for giving so many people freedom from their life threatening illness!"

"Yes, Sir," boomed Nambiar, punching the air with his thick index finger, "we should take-it-up with the government, Sir".

And on that note the meeting ended.

At the Transplant Center, the liver transplant operation on Kunju was in progress.

When the donor surgeon had first seen the liver at the donor hospital and called back to say that it looked good to go, Anesthetists had wheeled Kunju into the Operation Theater and started their work.

An iv line was started in one arm, and anesthesia begun. Kunju was soon asleep and would have no idea of the beehive of activity that erupted around him. With the ventilator taking over his breathing the Anesthetist was free to start putting in her 'lines'. The lines were numerous and of different types. There were short wide-bore lines into veins that would enable fast infusion of large volumes of fluids or blood. There were intravenous lines in the large jugular veins on both sides of the neck. Through the one on the right side a catheter was introduced that went straight down into the right side of the heart and then through its outflow tract, the pulmonary artery, into the lungs. The tip of this catheter, called a Swan Ganz catheter, floated in the pulmonary artery to give a continuous read out of the pressure there. When needed, a small transparent balloon near the tip could be inflated and catching the rush of blood in the pulmonary artery it would advance into a small branch of the pulmonary artery and wedge there to reflect the back pressure from the left side of the heart into which all blood from the lung must flow.

There were lines inserted into the arteries – one in the radial artery at the wrist, and another in the femoral artery in the groin. These were arterial lines. So critical is it to accurately measure the blood pressure, that not one but two lines – one from the top and one from the bottom half of the body – would be used to give a continuous read-out of the blood pressure throughout the operation. They would also be used to sample the blood going out from the heart to all the organs and tissues of the body, to check the level of oxygen it was carrying, and make sure that the acid and base composition was normal.

The gases entering Kunju's lungs and emerging from them were also being continuously monitored in the anesthetic machine. They would give the Anesthetist an idea of what the blood gases were. Checking blood samples and depending on the lab was a slower process meant to provide a reliable and documented cross-check.

The patient's own heart, lungs and kidneys, so extensively evaluated prior to listing him for transplant would usually be good enough to take him through the operation on their own steam. But if the kidneys failed they could be substituted with continuous dialysis throughout the operation; and the heart and lungs could, albeit rarely required, be assisted by an ECMO (extra corporeal membrane oxygenator) machine.

There is perhaps no operation with such profound physiological changes occurring during surgery as a liver transplant.

Removing the entire liver is itself a formidable surgical exercise in terms of the magnitude of trauma it can cause. Bleeding is part of any operation. What makes bleeding interesting during liver transplant is that blood clotting is mediated by factors (biological substances dissolved in the blood) that are produced in the liver. When the liver is diseased these factors are abnormally low, and the smallest wound can bleed to an extent that can be life threatening. Depending on the condition of the patient, and the extent to which his liver is defunct, the risk of serious hemorrhage has to be anticipated and prepared for. It is customary to arrange large quantities of blood, plasma, platelets and cryoprecipitate concentrates prior to a liver transplant operation. The Blood Bank gets ready to activate a massive transfusion protocol at short notice.

Once the diseased liver is removed, whatever little it could contribute to stop hemorrhage is also gone, and the anesthetist has to essentially keep the patient alive without his liver. There is no machine that can take over or reproduce the multiple functions of a human liver. In the case of a heart transplant also, the diseased heart had to be removed to make place for a new one, but during the time it took to complete the operation the patient could be kept alive by an artificial heart- lung machine that collected and oxygenated the blood coming into the heart, and pumped it to the body, fully oxygenated. There was no such option for the liver.

Artificial heart, lungs and kidneys have been developed and are in regular use, but there is no artificial liver available for clinical use. The anesthetist would just have to do whatever was possible to keep everything from going haywire. Monitoring the urine output and the function of the kidneys provided a good surrogate marker for the general state of body tissues and how they were functioning handling the stress of the operation. Assessing physiological needs, and anticipating them before they actually occurred was the skill of the liver transplant Anesthetist.

It would help to have a surgeon who did not do anything unpredictable. And most of all it would help to have a donor liver that would work the moment its blood supply was restored.

Although it is understood that surgeon and anesthetist work as a team, it is usually the case during a liver transplant operation that a surgeon has his hands full and his mind so completely occupied with the tasks he has to complete, that he is in no position to help the Anesthetist.

However experienced or hard-headed, no surgeon can completely ignore or suppress the visceral fear human beings have to the sight of blood. And when the blood is gushing it takes a stout heart and steady nerves to keep operating and perform the multiple complex steps that complete the operation. Initial attempts at liver transplant ended with the surgeons standing ankle deep in blood, and failure was attributed primarily to uncontrolled bleeding.

Further complicating blood loss in a liver transplant is the drastic reduction in blood flow back to the heart when the vessels entering the liver have to be clamped prior to removing the liver.

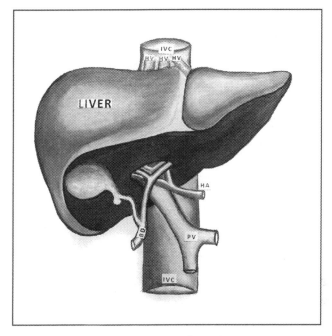

Line diagram of the liver

Fig 4: Line diagram of the liver.

BD= bile duct carrying bile from the liver to the intestine; PV= portal vein which brings blood from the intestines to the liver, carrying all the nutrients from food we eat to the liver to be processed before going to the heart via IVC for distribution all over the body; IVC= inferior vena cava which brings blood back to the heart from the lower half of the body, including the kidneys and lower limbs. It runs behind the liver receiving blood from the liver by small branches all along its course, and mainly from three large veins at the top of the liver called the hepatic veins (HV x 3).

During transplant the diseased liver has to be removed. The bile duct (BD) is divided, and hepatic artery (HA) and portal vein(PV) are clamped. The blood coming into the liver via the portal vein and hepatic artery is temporarily dammed up, and does not return to the heart. If the IVC is also required to be clamped to facilitate removal of the liver, blood return to the heart is even more profoundly reduced.

Before liver transplant could find wide application and go from being a project only for Superman, to an operation average human beings could be trained to accomplish, it had to be done "on bypass". This process involved using a pump that collected blood from the intestines (via the portal vein), and the lower body (via the inferior vena cava) and transferred this around the liver to the upper body enabling it to flow (via cannulas in the jugular vein or the axillary vein) into the heart. The veno-venous bypass pump allowed liver transplant to become safer for the patient, and easier on surgeons and anesthetists. The complex portions of the operation did not require to be rushed, and could be mastered by surgeons in training.

Additionally, several innovations in electrocautery machines made it easier to stop bleeding from large raw surfaces that result when the liver is taken out of the body leaving a gaping hole in the upper abdomen. Developed in the 1980s and still popular with liver transplant surgeons, is the 'argon beam coagulator'. Someone discovered that a jet of argon will conduct electricity. Directed at a bleeding vessel the argon jet blows away the blood and exposes the bleeding point that is coagulated by the electric current shooting down the high pressure jet of argon. The crackle and smoke, the bright arcing flame of the argon beam make it look like a welder at work.

What remains after the argon has been blasted at bleeding tissue is a charred expanse. A trainee surgeon's natural proclivity to ration the argon beam and limit the burn is dismissed by the aphorism, "if it looks black, then it is probably not red.". No deleterious effects of such charring have been discovered.

The argon beam turned out not to be the final solution for bleeding during a liver transplant. Different materials that would cause blood to clot by alternative means have been developed. They ranged from pieces of gauze-like 'surgicel', to sponge like 'gel-foam' to wool-like 'fibrillar collagen'. There were also synthetically prepared liquid concentrates of clotting factors that could be sprayed under pressure onto bleeding surfaces. They were supposed to cause blood to clot even where clotting factors were deficient.

For times when surgery had to continue without pause and never mind the bleeding, machines had been developed that would collect the blood, separate red cells, wash them of whatever might have contaminated them in the surgical field, and reinfuse the blood back to the patient. The machine was called, aptly, a 'cell saver'.

Saved cells, and packed red cells from the blood bank would be stored in the reservoir of a 'rapid infusion device'. Also called 'the Belmont' it had been designed by its manufacturer "for high volume infusion during surgery … in trauma and on the battlefield". At the touch of a button, blood could be pumped into the body at rates of upto a liter a minute, and the machine employed electromagnetic induction heating to get the blood up to body temperature as it rushed in, thus preventing fatal hypothermia.

When large volumes of fluid were moving in and out of the body, it was inevitable that body temperature would drop. This could make bleeding worse, and cause profound derangements, including acid build up and cardiac arrest. So important is it to keep the patient's temperature normal or near normal that multiple devices are employed during a liver transplant for this purpose. The operation table has a special warming blanket on which the patient is placed, through which circulates warm water via a pump and thermostat. Covering him were air-circulating blankets called 'Bair huggers' that blew in hot air into the conducting channels that hugged the patient close. Core body temperature would be monitored throughout the operation by a special transducer connected to a thermistor device in the catheter inserted into the patient's bladder. Thus both urine output and core body temperature could be monitored via the same catheter.

Wrapped around his legs were compression pumps, called Sequential Compression Devices(SCDs), that would keep periodically compressing and releasing his calf muscles to help with circulation in the peripheries of his legs, and prevent blood clots from forming in them through the long operation.

All of these devices, gadgets and monitors had one thing in common: they were very expensive and easily broken.

In addition, the machines required specialized personnel to operate them. In a complex case the patient would be surrounded by a small horde of cell-saver technicians, pump technicians, dialysis personnel in addition to anesthesia techs, circulating nurses, blood bank personnel trying not to trample each other in the operating room as surgeons and anesthetists struggled, the atmosphere grew tense and a patient's life could hang by a thread.

Before Dr. A scrubbed in on the operation, he went over to the adjacent operating room where the donor surgeon had unwrapped the bags in which he had transported the liver from the donor hospital, packed in ice. The liver now lay in a basin in a pool of bloodstained preservation fluid in its sterile bag, surrounded by ice. The amount of blood in the fluid would give Dr. A an idea of how the donor operation had gone. The less he saw, the happier he would be, though he had no scientifically valid proof on which to base such optimism.

More importantly, he checked the labels on the box used to transport the liver, and looked at the paperwork that had accompanied the organ, checking the blood group. Although this had been done multiple times in the course of the whole transplant coordination activity by coordinators, nurses, and even by other surgeons, the final check was his responsibility.

This was also the last point in time at which he could call a halt to the operation if something did not look right.

Today, everything was looking good. The preservation fluid in the bags was not too bloody. The liver itself looked excellent. It was a dark healthy tan color, not the sickly red or frank yellow that indicated excess fat in the liver. More importantly, it had sharp edges, and was not enlarged.

Peering over the shoulder of his colleague who had done the organ retrieval, he looked at the 'hilum' – the area in the middle of the liver, recessed from the front edge, where major blood vessels enter the liver, and the bile duct emerges.

"Artery?" he asked.

The donor surgeon selected a fine vascular forceps from the array set out on the backtable, and gently lifted the artery. He had brought back the entire artery all the way from the aorta. Branches to the stomach, spleen and pancreas had required to be divided on the way, and he displayed the anatomy and each branch. This was also, in essence, a demonstration of how good a job he had done.

"Single artery", he answered pointing it out, adding, unnecessarily, "no damage".

"Looks good," Dr. A said approvingly, and went out of the room.

There was perhaps another half an hour of work remaining to be done, he estimated, to prepare the liver to be implanted into the recipient. He had to get going with the operation on Kunju. No time to waste.

Finding the senior nurse in charge of the OT, he said, "We are proceeding. Please send word to the Aliyar Kunju family."

The nurse nodded happily, and left to find the family in the waiting area. She always told them to go back to their room and wait for word from her. She would call into the room and give them a regular update on how things were going. She knew how hard it is to have to wait and have no news as the clock ticked, and time seemed to stretch to eternity.

After showing the artery to his Chief, the donor surgeon turned the liver around in the basin. The water was freezing, and his fingers were chilled to the bone. He would have to ignore the cold and work with frozen fingers while completing the preparation of the liver.

Starting at the back of the liver he worked on the short length of the IVC that was closely attached to the liver. Numerous branches from the liver entered the IVC, and he would have to judiciously tie those that were not helpful to the process of implantation, while preserving the important ones. Next, he worked on the portal vein that brings blood from the intestines and other digestive organs into the liver. This delicate vein had to be carefully separated from the fat and other tissues surrounding it. He would also be freeing it from the more slender, but thicker walled hepatic artery. The portal vein required the freedom so it could to be sewed to the portal vein of the recipient, aligning the two to conform to the Geometric definition of a straight line: the shortest distance between two points.

He then cleaned off all unnecessary tissues and fat surrounding the liver, and removed the attached muscular diaphragm that he had taken along with the liver to protect the capsule while removing it from the donor's body.

Last of all, the hepatic artery was dissected. This runs a long course from the aorta, supplying branches to the stomach, pancreas and duodenum, before it becomes exclusive to the liver. Carefully ligating the branches that were not needed, taking care that the actual artery was not distorted, and its delicate inner lining membrane called the intima, was not stretched or cracked, the artery was prepared as the final step of the backtable procedure. Although the donor surgeon would preserve the artery in its entire length, the actual length used in the recipient operation would depend on what the surgeon operating in the next room found as he, equally meticulously, dissected the hepatic artery in the recipient.

When the procedure was complete, and the liver was ready to be implanted into the recipient, it was returned to the sterile bags in which it had been initially packed and transported, adding fresh ice to the basin in which it would be kept in the recipient OR.

When he left the room in which the liver was being prepared, Dr. A, Chief liver transplant surgeon, had moved to the room where the recipient operation was underway on Kunju.

He opened a small rectangular wooden box he was carrying in which his surgical 'loupes': magnifying glasses, were stored. They would enlarge the image of whatever he was looking at by two and a half times. The glasses were custom made for him based on the precise distance between his pupils, and the depth at which he personally liked to operate. Mounted on black old-fashioned frame spectacles, the magnifying lenses projected from the front like two miniature telescopes. Encircling his head he strapped the circular band of a headlight that projected from the middle of his forehead sending out a powerful beam of cold white light which he focused onto his hands. Whatever he now focused on through the telescopes would be brightly illuminated. The powerful overhead operating lights, sufficient to operate on the surface and also within a body cavity would not suffice at the depth to which he planned on going. He jiggled the light and his glasses tightening the straps on each till he was satisfied they would not move while he was operating. He focused on his palms and fingertips till the individual creases were blown up into serpentine ridges and valleys.

The Transplant Fellow who was assisting the Chief on this case had already opened the abdomen. Scrubbed in with him were a senior scrub nurse and her junior assistant nurse. The electrocautery machine whined as subcutaneous tissue and muscles were cut with the electric current and hemostasis secured.

Unlike the donor operation, opening the abdomen in the recipient is a time consuming process. Large dilated veins, similar to the ones in the esophagus that had bled and almost exsanguinated Kunju when he first realized he had cirrhosis, were present in other tissues as well. In the subcutaneous fat concealed under the skin they lay waiting to bleed torrentially when divided. They were of course much easier to see and control than veins in the esophagus.

Once the abdomen was opened a suction tube with oversheath guard was introduced into the abdomen to remove the collected fluid. About 4 liters gushed out almost instantaneously and filled the suction bottle near the side wall of the operating room. More was present in the recesses of Kunju's abdomen, and even more would form as the case went on. This was just another manifestation of increased pressure in the abdominal veins that drain towards the liver where blood was backed up due to high resistance from the scar tissue that had replaced the liver.

The scarred liver was soon visible to all in the operating room. It was misshapen, with odd bulges and ugly greenish excrescences on its surface. It sat in a pool of yellowish brown fluid like a hump backed toad in a puddle. All around it were thick dilated veins, and the peritoneal membrane lining the inside of the abdomen, normally white with a fine skein of capillary sized vessels, was beefy red and angry looking. Everything was waiting to spew forth blood when touched.

Dr. A and the Transplant Fellow put in the abdominal retractor to open up the cave in which the liver lay. The overlying ribcage had to be lifted up and out of the way. The right kidney stuck to the liver below had to be separated from it and retracted downwards. Stomach and loops of intestine had to be moved away from the vicinity of the liver. Soon the incision, made in the shape of an inverted Y, was surrounded by bars and blades of stainless steel converting it into a massive gaping hole. Flat paddle like blades inserted into the abdomen would keep everything away from the liver to which attention would be directed for the rest of the operation. The steel retractor system, which cost as much as a small car, would perform actions previously delegated to three assistants who invariably, unsteadily, grew more and more weary as the operation progressed. With the fancy retractor systems it was possible now to do the operation with only one assistant. There was a lot less heartburn and cussing, and transplants got done more efficiently.

The Recipient operation of a liver transplant was divided into three distinct phases:

- Hepatectomy, when the diseased liver was removed, cutting through blood vessels and tissue attachments to mobilize the liver and remove it.
- Anhepatic phase, when the liver was out, and there was enough exposure within the large cave that remained, to get hemostasis done
- Implant, when the new liver was sewn in, and circulation re-established.

Dr. A planned to do the whole operation "off bypass", dispensing with the system of tubes and pump that diverted blood around the liver, as was standard practice in the past. He had, over the years, developed the necessary speed and skill to get through the period when all blood return to the heart from the abdomen and lower body was interrupted. His team of anesthetists had also learned to manage without the bypass.

The 'ligaments' or connecting tissues that anchored the liver to the diaphragm were first divided, taking care to identify and control all bleeding vessels that run through these structures. Some could just be burned through with the electrocautery or the argon beam coagulator. Others were too large for this, and required to be sutured. On the left side the spleen had to be protected from injury. On the right, the kidney and the right adrenal gland were separated from the liver. The right adrenal gland stuck to, and reluctant to part with its lifelong neighbor had to be prised away. Dr. A, unwilling to give it much respect, managed to shred it, fit only to be subsequently cauterized to a crisp.

He was eager to get quickly to the hilum of the liver where he would locate and divide bile duct, hepatic artery, and portal vein in that order. Maximum available lengths of each of these structures were preserved. The hepatic artery was carefully dissected back to the point where it gave off its final branches to duodenum and pancreas before becoming exclusively the artery to the liver. The junction of hepatic artery and its final large branch to the duodenum could, if he wanted, later be used for joining the donor artery. The portal vein now came into view. With overlying artery and bile duct stripped away, it stretched blue and turgid between the liver and the pancreas. Applying a fine vascular clamp across its base, Dr. A divided it as high as possible. Later, he knew, he would trim much of it away, but for now, the more the merrier.

Disconnected from all that gave it significance, the liver now only had to be lifted off the inferior vena cava (IVC), the largest vein in the human body which lay behind it. This was sooner said than done. Running from the back of the liver and directly into the IVC were a variable number of small and delicate veins. They had no useful function in normal life and were Mother Nature's back up system in case the three major veins at the top of the liver, the major channels returning blood from liver to heart, should get occluded. Though not large, the short hepatic veins would bleed if accidentally torn, or if a ligature slipped, and this bleeding would then be occurring at the deepest part of the human body.

Dr. A proceeded carefully and very very respectfully, ligating each vein twice, before dividing it, inching his way up the back of the liver and separating it from the IVC. The Anesthetist, knowing the danger of the area where he was working, kept the pressure in the IVC low, so that if a ligature slipped or a vein was inadvertently torn, the surgeons would have some chance of getting it under control without exsanguinating the patient.

The operation slowed, and the room became silent. People spoke in whispers so nothing would distract the surgeon. It was like a Wimbledon final before the second serve at match-point. Nobody breathes unless they absolutely must.

The liver came off the cava, and finally there were only the three major hepatic veins at the top, barely visible under the diaphragm. He was unable to actually see them, but Dr. A knew they were there. Putting a curved vascular clamp across the left and middle veins, and firing a stapler across the right, he removed the liver, hefting its weight with both hands into a large basin for the ugly specimen to be taken off the field and packed off to Pathology.

The patient was now 'anhepatic': he was alive, without a liver.

No pool of blood welled up in the gaping hole where the liver had once lived, no noisy whirring of multiple suckers, no cursing at bleeders refusing to stop bleeding. Things were going well today, the Anesthetist noted, peeking over the top of the drape stretched across the patient separating her from the surgeons and the operative field. She liked to call it the 'blood-brain barrier' punning on the physiological structure that, within the skull, protected delicate brain cells from noxious substances in the blood stream.

She was, of course, the delicate brain cell. The surgeon, bloody and sweating on the other side, was the noxious substance.

She sent off a set of labs, drawing blood which would go to the Blood Gas lab and others to the main Hematology and Chemistry labs downstairs. Another sample was drawn for the Thromboelastograph (TEG)

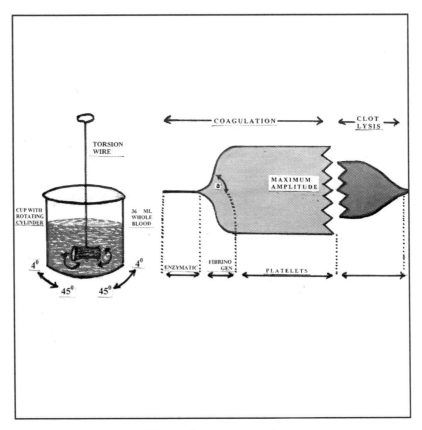

Thromboelastograph

Fig 5: Thromboelastograph (TEG).

The image on the left shows the basics of the TEG machine. On the right is the TEG tracing obtained.

Procedure: A small amount of blood (36 ml) is placed into a cup in which a cylinder rotates. As the blood clots the rotating cylinder encounters increasing resistance. The resistance to rotation is transferred via the torsion wire, to a recording paper. When the blood is liquid initially the tracing is a straight line. As the blood clots the resistance increases and the graph becomes wide. The actual clotting process can be studied in this manner (see labels of different phases of the graph)

Use: Bleeding during liver transplant is a major problem. The TEG helps anesthetists decide what exactly is required to restore the ability of blood to clot and stop the bleeding while the surgeon is taking out the old liver and sewing in the new liver.

Although the TEG would take much longer to complete, she would know in a short time from the initial tracing if she needed to be giving the patient fresh frozen plasma or other blood products.

Today it did not look like too much would be required.

Dr. A glanced at the clock in the operating room, silently calculating the cold ischemia time: the time the liver had been sitting on ice after being removed from the body of the donor.

Sometime in the future, perhaps, they would find a better way to preserve organs, and the liver would be kept warm and oxygenated, with blood flowing, bile being formed, and all other functions intact while the recipient operation proceeded at a safe and leisurely pace. Now however, speed was of the essence. In theory he could take upto 12 hours, and the liver would still eventually work. In practice, the shorter the cold ischemia time, the better the chances the liver would work right away, and the organs that depended on it would remain undamaged. Perhaps most importantly, after the operation was done, everything would be working fine, and he and the rest of his team, would have a hope of getting some rest.

Bringing the ice-cold basin containing the liver onto the operating field, and unwrapping the three sterile bags in which it was contained, the scrub nurse marked the beginning of the third and final phase of the liver transplant: the Implant.

"Liver out of ice. Note the time," ordered Dr. A. From this point on till blood flow was restored into the new liver the time taken had to be minimal. In theory the liver was best kept cold until blood flow was restored, and to help it stay that way while the vessels were sutured together, the nurse would keep irrigating it with cold saline to try and negate the rise in surface temperature caused by contact with the warm body the liver would be nestled in.

There are few if any operations today that require speed. Improvements in Anesthesia have made it unnecessary for a surgeon to be quick. Transplant surgery is the one exception to that rule, and during a transplant operation, it is this phase of the operation – actually sewing in the new organ, attaching its blood vessels – that has to be done as quickly as possible.

It is also the most delicate part of the operation. It is the part of the operation that most powerfully influences the eventual success or failure of the transplant. For a surgeon, the emphasis has to shift from excising an organ – always a bloody process bordering on butchery – to performing a needle-and-thread job that even the finest, most accomplished seamstress, with all week at her disposal, would find demanding.

Surgeons in training are taught, in an attempt to promote meticulousness over speed, that a fast surgeon is one who does not have to repeat steps or redo an operation. The sewing process for a transplant surgeon has to be done perfectly if it is to be done quickly. It has to be right the first time. Having to redo a vascular anastomosis, is the worst thing that can happen to a transplant surgeon. In his mind, it is not an option.

Vascular anastomosis was once regarded so technically difficult, that they actually gave a Nobel Prize to the person, Alexis Carrel, 1912, who showed it could be done. No Nobel Prize has ever before or since been given for something so prosaic as a stitching technique.

The organ being sewn in is also not a natural fit for the recipient. It can be too large or too small depending on the size of the donor. Its shape, which is normal, is completely different from the shape of the organ it is replacing. Neighboring structures that have molded and accomodated over years to a misshapen diseased organ can sometimes intrude and make it difficult to seat the new liver in the place of the old one.

The length to which each blood vessel has to be trimmed before it is sutured is a matter of judgment – the surgeon's visual approximation of the best fit. Whether he got it right or not would be known only when blood flow is restored. Kinks, narrowing, redundancy, or twists can occur. When flow within the blood vessel is turbulent, it will clot.

A clotted blood vessel is a dead structure.

When flow is pulsatile, as in an artery, it can result in the vessel whiplashing around furiously like a garden hose to which the tap has suddenly been turned on. In their natural condition blood vessels are immobile structures, surrounded by elastic tissue that tuck the vessel snugly in its bed, while accommodating the expansion, relaxation, or contraction associated with changes in flow. These supporting tissues have, of necessity been shredded in the course of explanting the liver from the donor's body. Suturing a blood vessel requires it to be stripped of its surrounding tissue anyway, and the extent to which this is done during a transplant has to be kept to a minimum even if that makes it difficult to see and sew.

Lastly, in the context of a transplant as opposed to regular vascular surgery, the tissue quality of the blood vessel is completely different on the two sides of the suture line. On the donor's side blood vessels are healthy, resilient and tenacious. On the recipient's side they can be swollen, friable, and diseased. Sutures that slide well on one side can cut through on the other leaving a jagged, frayed margin that is hard to work with the second time around should redoing a suture line become absolutely necessary.

The first vascular anastomosis performed in a liver transplant is to establish outflow from the liver. There were two ways this could be accomplished: the older American way where the donor IVC at the top of the liver would be sutured to a common cuff of the recipient's hepatic veins end-to-end; or the more recent French modification, in which the IVC of donor and recipient were sutured together side-to side. The former was more anatomically proper and it did not require clamping and interrupting flow through the IVC while doing the suturing. The latter was typically French – a cheeky innovation that, like a Debussy roulade, had completely changed the melody and measure of how surgeons constructed hepatic outflow during liver transplant.

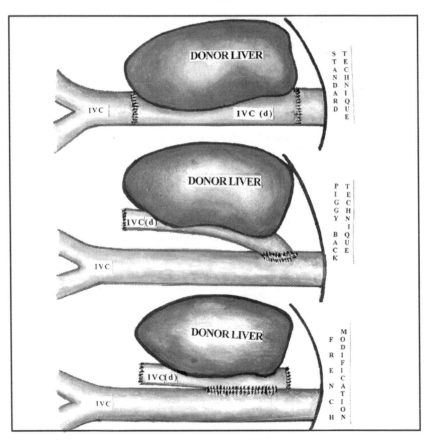

**Fig 6: Diagram to show different techniques
of implantation of the donor liver.**

In the standard technique the diseased liver of the recipient is removed along with the segment of inferior vena cava (IVC) which is closely applied to it. The donor liver along with its own IVC(d) is implanted into the space replacing the segment of IVC removed along with the recipient's diseased liver.

The piggy-back technique retains the entire IVC of the recipient, carefully taking the diseased liver off the IVC and ligating the small branches that run to it from the liver. The donor liver is placed on top of the IVC – hence the name 'piggy-back' for this modification. The IVC(d) is anastomosed to the recipient at the upper end close to the heart.

The French modification of the piggy-back technique is done by a long side-to-side anastomosis between the recipient IVC and IVC(d) after closing off the upper and lower ends of IVC(d).

Dr. A took the donor liver out of the ice, and dropped it gently into the hole where Kunju's liver once lay. It settled awkwardly, crumpling under its own weight into the hollow above the kidney where the abdominal cavity was deepest. Grabbing the left lobe he brought the liver forward and stretched it, seeing if he could line up the IVC of donor and recipient. It lined up nearly perfectly for Kunju, and the size match looked perfect. This liver would be suitable to hook up by either American or French technique. This patient was looking lucky, Dr. A said to himself. He decided to go with the older American technique, and not clamp the IVC at all.

The first sutures were placed aligning the corners. The backwall was then sutured with a running technique carefully tightening each throw so that it was not tight enough to crumple the sutures or cause a purse-string narrowing effect, while not allowing any gaps through which bleeding would occur at the back of the liver. This was an area where it is almost impossible to see properly to put in additional stitches to get control of bleeding. Once the back was completed satisfactorily, the front or anterior wall of the vein was much more easily sutured, and the anastomosis establishing outflow was complete.

Next, the inflow into the liver was addressed. Before starting suturing, Dr. A flushed out the liver using albumin infused into the liver via the portal vein. It flowed into the liver and ran out from the lower end of the donor IVC. The objective was to flush out the preservative fluid contained in the liver, and any other stuff accumulated while it was kept in ice. When the albumin flush was completed, the lower end of the donor IVC would be sutured shut. Anything flowing from the liver into the IVC would now go up towards the upper end, and enter the right atrium of the heart.

Dr. A was now ready to start sewing the portal vein and the hepatic artery.

Unlike other organs, the liver is unique in that it has a dual inflow: the artery, called the hepatic artery, brings oxygenated blood from the heart, and the portal vein brings blood from the intestines and other abdominal organs. Of the two, it was by far the portal vein which carried more blood. In a normal individual the inflow was 80% from the portal vein, and 20% from the hepatic artery. In someone with cirrhosis, the portal vein flow was huge, much more than the normal. How the new liver would handle the massively increased inflow only time would tell. What was important now was to see that the vessels were joined perfectly, minimizing the risk of occlusion or clotting.

The portal veins of donor and recipient were the first to be connected. Below, on the recipient side, the portal vein was about double the diameter of the donor portal vein above. The combined length of donor and recipient portal veins was also excessive. Carefully trimming the excess length was necessary before starting to suture. Trim too little and the vein would be floppy. Too much, and it would stretch and tear apart when the blood flowed in and engorged the now empty vessel. After making a V-shaped cut on the donor side to increase its effective diameter, suturing was begun.

"Ready to unclamp in five minutes!", Dr. A called out to the Anesthetists. They would need all hands on deck when clamps were released. All hell could break loose when blood flow was restored to the liver, and it rushed through it to the heart.

Toxic products of cellular metabolism are regularly released into the blood stream all the time, all over the body. The rate at which this occurs is normally slow enough for protective 'homeostatic' systems to handle the load. When tissues are deprived of blood, however, toxins accumulate, and when blood flow is restored these toxic substances come flooding back into circulation. Blood levels of potassium can rise high enough to arrest the heart. In the specific context of a liver transplant, these unnamed products of cellular ischemia, this potassium load, directly gush into the right side of the heart with no opportunity of prior dilution, thus greatly increasing the chance of cardiac arrest.

In addition, there are substances, not all known, that come out of the ischemic liver, and moving through the right side of the heart, enter and cause a precipitous rise in pulmonary artery pressure. The pulmonary artery is the only outflow tract of the right heart. If it shuts down, blood backs up acutely into the right side of the heart, and no blood reaches either the lungs or the left side of the heart that pumps to all structures, organs and tissues in the body. This effectively results in circulatory arrest, synonymous with death.

The anesthetist had to prepare for all these events. Adequate levels of bicarbonate and calcium in the blood could protect the heart from the effects of high potassium. The machine used to shock the heart if it arrests was fired up and primed to go into action and jump start the heart if required. Blood pressure and blood volume were optimized to normal or near normal so that the effect of a transient drop in blood pressure would be minimized.

The Anesthetist checked and rechecked everything to make sure she was ready.

Delicate brain cell she might be, but at this time she had to have a stout heart and steady nerves. There was very little the surgeon could do to help her to deal with disaster.

The anastomosis of the portal vein was quickly completed. At the end the knot was tied very loose in a technique called the 'growth factor', invented by Thomas Starzl, the first person to have accomplished a liver transplant successfully. The loose suture line could result in some bleeding when flow was restored through it, but this technique would avoid a narrowing at this site in future as the smaller donor portal vein grew in diameter as it learned to accommodate the abnormally high inflow from the recipient vein.

It was time to reperfuse Mohamed Aliyar Kunju's new liver.

The clamp on the IVC was first opened establishing the outflow from the liver. Some blood flowed back into the liver, and a patchy color change from grey-brown to dark red was seen. Dr. A looked quickly at the suture line at the top of the liver, the area most difficult to see and access. He was relieved to see that his technique had been good, and there was no obvious bleeding.

The most critical time during the reperfusion had come. With one eye on the overhead monitors, and another on the portal vein, Dr. A gingerly released the clamp on the portal vein. The rush of blood was like a water hammer. It bulged the portal vein, whipping it into life, ruthlessly distending it, stretching and tearing at the fresh suture line like some medieval torture ritual. The color change in the liver was breathtaking, as a red blush spread throughout the liver. The liver as a whole also swelled visibly as its blood volume was restored. Dr. A kept his hand on the surface of the liver, caressing it, comforting it, as it convulsed mightily back to life. He was also feeling it for undue tension that could indicate a problem with the outflow – either at the suture line, or beyond it within Kunju's heart and lungs – causing blood to back up within the liver. The liver capsule, tough and resilient and able normally to withstand considerable pressure, has been known to crack open under the combined influence of high inflow and poor outflow resulting in torrential bleeding.

This did not happen today.

Dr. A was also satisfied by the appearance of the portal vein after it had filled. The donor portal vein had stretched to double its original size, but there was no narrowing at the suture line. With no angulation or redundancy, donor and recipient veins were keeping a straight line.

The EKG tracing, on the other hand should *not* become a straight line! Anesthetist and surgeon were both happy with the way it stayed steady, squiggly, with normal rhythmic upstrokes corresponding to pulses on the arterial tracing. The blood pressure dropped transiently, then held steady. Kunju's heart was good.

After five or ten minutes while the nurse bathed the liver in hot saline, encouraging it now to return to body temperature, and everybody watched to see that the patient stayed stable, the surgeon was ready to continue the operation.

In the old days this was the time to take a break and have a cigarette. Nicotine can help bring down the anxiety level. It may also bring down soaring testosterone to comfortable levels. Nobody justified such breaks any more, and most surgeons no longer smoked. Their high testosterone levels had either found other ways to scale down, or perhaps they did not peak any longer as they used to when liver transplant was regarded as the equivalent of a Formula One car race, and pitt-stops were part of the circuit.

After a quick round of hemostasis, Dr. A continued without a break straight on to suturing the artery. Although the artery carries only 20% of total blood flow into the liver, it brings most of the oxygen. Structures within the liver that are highly dependent on this oxygen can suffer irreversible damage if the hepatic artery blood supply is found wanting. The most sensitive of all are the bile ducts. Without a good hepatic arterial supply, bile ducts within the liver shrivel up, scar down, form strictures, and in places dilate into lakes of stagnant bile. Stagnant bile, like stagnant water, soon becomes putrid. The infection that occurs in the liver can break its confines and spread into the blood resulting in septicemia.

Biliary infection and septicemia are bad news in any individual. In someone taking medications that suppress the immune system to prevent rejection it can be quickly fatal. For those who somehow survive the infection, re-transplantation is the only treatment option.

Dr. A had earlier dissected Kunju's hepatic artery back until he found the branch to the duodenum and stomach, and now decided to utilize the junction to create a large opening which he used to join the donor artery. A larger diameter at the site of the anastomosis, would hopefully minimize the risk of clot formation within the artery and the train of biliary complications described above that he tried not to think about at this time.

More hemostasis followed, carefully inspecting all areas where blood could be seen, and controlling the bleeding. The argon beam coagulator, the bi-polar electrocautery, gellfoam packs, surgical packs, everything that was required and available was used to get the operating field dry and all bleeding under control.

Sometimes during a liver transplant, hemostasis - controlling the bleeding - takes as much time as all the other steps combined. It is a painstaking chore, the apogee of drudgery for an exhausted surgical team.

Only when the liver looked well perfused, and no blood visible anywhere it shouldn't be seen, did Dr. A take a break. His assistants would also take short breaks.

Scrub nurses, better able to hold their bladders, generally didn't take a break till the end of their shift when they would hand over to the next set of nurses and leave. The captains and the kings had gone, the tumult and the shouting was ended. Left temporarily to their own devices, they started a preliminary count of instruments, sponges, and gauze pieces. The nurses coming in to replace them would want the count to have been done and everything accounted for. Nothing could be left behind at the end of the operation.

The final structure to be connected was the bile duct. The surgeons returned. First the gall bladder of the donor liver was removed, and the donor and recipient bile ducts were measured off, trimmed, and sutured together. Although this anastomosis was the least stressful, it was called the Achilles' heel of a liver transplant. Over the next few days, as the liver began to produce more bile, the slimy fluid could leak between sutures that looked adequate now with bile ducts empty. Strictures could happen, and above a stricture the bile duct would dilate. Liver function tests immediately reflect abnormalities in bile flow, but it is hard to be sure that is the only reason. Rejection, the result of the immune system attacking the liver also affects bile ducts, and to differentiate the two a biopsy is necessary. The treatment of the two conditions is very different and a mistaken diagnosis can have serious consequences to the patient.

With the bile duct complete and looking satisfactory, another round of hemostasis was undertaken. Kunju's new liver was gently maneuvered from side to side, and from back to front as every cranny and crevice in the area was checked. If blood had collected somewhere a search was made for the source of hemorrhage.

Finally the entire field was irrigated with an antibiotic solution. Drains were placed to siphon out any blood, bile or ascites fluid that might collect even after all possible precautions had been taken for none of this to happen, and the abdomen was closed.

They say that Murphy, of 'Murphy's law' fame, was an aircraft maintenance mechanic. Anything that could go wrong, he had proclaimed, *would* go wrong.

Transplant surgeons believe Murphy was an optimist. In this business things go wrong that cannot, possibly, ever, go wrong.

No other operation is as unforgiving of error as a liver transplant.

Part IV

RECOVERY

Waiting is always difficult.

After having waited so long to be called in for the transplant, waiting for the operation to get done seemed to be the hardest part for Ayesha. Shehnaz and Raza had arrived about 3 hours after Kunju had been wheeled into the Operation Theater. They sat with her in the private room allotted to them, and waited for the phone to ring with news from the OT. Ayesha could not bear to pick up the phone, and Shehnaz had taken over that function. Raza alternately paced the floor and sat playing with his iPhone. Mother and daughter spoke quietly about home things, relatives, and what they were variously doing. Shehnaz called a few of the relatives that they knew Kunju would want to inform and told them Dad was in surgery.

Dinner time came and went. Nobody was feeling hungry. Closer to midnight, Raza said he wanted to have a snack, before the hospital cafeteria closed. Not wanting to be separated, they picked up their personal things and left the room telling the nurse at the desk to call them if there was word from the OT.

At the cafeteria, Ayesha recognized Krishnan's wife sitting in a corner. She went over to speak with her, and then came back to the table where Shehnaz and Raza were sitting with their coffee and sandwiches.

"Guess what! Krish is getting his kidney transplant as well. He is also in the OT now. He must have matched with the same donor whose liver is being transplanted into your Dad!"

"Really? Wow!" Shehnaz and Raza said excitedly. "What are the odds of that happening? Two people meet in hospital, waiting for their transplants, and end up with the same donor!"

"They have taken him into the OT. The matching process only just got done," said Ayesha. She then explained the difference between the matching process for kidney and liver that she had learned earlier that day.

"Wow, Mom!" Shehnaz said admiringly, "you know so much about all this now! You can become an advisor to people who need a transplant!"

Ayesha blushed. She was not accustomed to being praised for her knowledge by her children who had much more education than she ever got.

When they got back to their ward room, the nurse at the front desk said that OT had called to say Kunju would be shifted to the ICU in another hour or so. The operation was over, and they could go down to the Conference Room outside the OT and where the surgeon would come out and talk to them.

They raced off to meet the surgeon.

Dr. A was not looking like Asterix the great and indomitable Gaul warrior he was named after. He looked, rather, like he was in serious need of some magic potion. He was sitting in the conference room in his surgical scrubs, with crumpled cap and his mask dangling over his shirt-front like a baby's bib. He was waiting for them, and appeared to have dozed off when they opened door and walked in. It was past 2 AM.

"Just finished the operation," he said without ceremony or preamble, "it went well."

He made it sound like there was not much more to be said. The three family members who had rushed to meet him stood in a line staring at him. He sat looking up at them and sleepily blinked once, twice. Ayesha, so habituated to reading between lines, was thrown off at getting only one line and therefore nothing to read between. She was at a loss as to what to say. She glanced at Raza, hoping he would ask something. He looked like he had heard whatever he needed to hear. How useless can guys be? Ayesha fumed silently.

Shehnaz was the first to collect her wits.

"Is he out of the operating room, Doctor?" she asked brightly, "can we see him?"

"Yes and No," he replied enigmatically, waking up a bit with her energetic voice. "Yes, he is out of the operating room and back in the ICU, but No, you cannot see him just yet. The nurses have to get everything settled with his iv lines and fluids and drains and monitors etc., only then they will let you know you can come and see him. He has to look presentable before you can go see him."

'Presentable' was a misnomer for what they saw when they finally got to see Kunju. Dawn was breaking outside the window of their room, before the nurse at the desk came to tell them they could go down to the ICU.

At the entrance under the stern eye of the senior nurse, they had to wash their hands in an alcohol based scrub-solution, wear a cap and mask and full-length green gown before entering the ICU.

They were allowed in only one at a time. They had to get back to their room upstairs, before they could compare their observations.

"Oh God, he looks awful!" exclaimed Ayesha.

"Good thing they did not let us in to see him earlier. Remember, this is after he has been made to look presentable!" said Raza.

"How can you be so calm and detached? He's your father. You should be the one to go and tell the doctors he doesn't look right."

"But, Mom, you heard the nurses tell you he is doing fine!"

"How can you believe them? Did you even look at him while you were there?" Ayesha was mad at her son and determined to scold him for whatever she thought was not going right.

"What do you think, Shehnaz?" he asked helplessly. Diffusing the brunt of maternal attack by collective sibling force, was a strategy he had long practiced.

"I think we should stop arguing, and just each one keep a diary record of what we think", said the ever resourceful Shehnaz. "That way we will not be arguing and blaming each other, and we will have a nice little record of what we saw and how we feel. Right now, I agree with Mom, he does look pretty dreadful. But if the nurses say he is OK they are probably right. They have seen many more cases than we have."

Kunju's dreadful appearance was mostly the result of the large amount of fluid given during surgery, and the fact that this was most evident on his face. He was asleep, sedated, the nurse had said, and the ventilator at his bedside was hooked up to a tube in his mouth. Shehnaz had asked what it was, and the nurse had told her it was an 'endotracheal tube', going into his trachea and letting the machine do the breathing for him. And the tube in his nose? It was going into his stomach, keeping it decompressed. Under his sheets there were three tubes coming out of his belly, attached to suction bottles of transparent plastic. Only Shehnaz had seen these.

"How did you find out they were there?" asked Ayesha.

"Oh I went to hold his hand, and suddenly there was this warm thing pressing on my hand, gave me such a fright! I moved his sheets a little and looked at it. It was full of blood! I got such a shock I almost screamed! Then the nurse showed me the drain. There were two on the right side and one on the left. Everyone gets three of them, it seems."

"You held his hand? How did they let you do that? Nobody is supposed to touch him!" Ayesha was horrified.

"Oh Ma, why would they ask you to scrub your hands with alcohol if you are not allowed to touch him?" asked Shehnaz with compelling logic.

"He will get some infection!"

"He'll be fine!"

Mother and daughter glared at each other.

Raza tried to diffuse the crisis.

"I liked the nurse", he said, satisfied, "I think she is pretty cute."

And then when both mother and sister transferred their glares to him, he added hastily, "I mean, I think she will look after Dad just fine. We just need to let her do her thing. I think Shehnaz has a great idea. Let's just stop arguing and write our diaries. And we will compare them after Dad gets home, and that way he also will know whatever happened. I mean, he has no idea right now what is going on. Right? I mean, he is totally unconscious, so ......?"

Shehnaz's diary.

Today is the first day of Dad's new liver.

They call it Day 0, as in zero. I asked them why it was not Day #1, but they said the operation finished in the early hours this morning, so today is still the day of the operation, not yesterday when they took him into the operating room. Whatever.

Anyway, Dad looks pretty awful. I don't know what they did to him, but I can barely recognize him. His face is so swollen, his eyelids look like he wouldn't be able to open them. He is asleep so it probably doesn't matter.

There are tubes all over. They come out of his neck and face and belly. The nurses have to keep track of all of them, and what is going in and coming out is all carefully measured and recorded. They have so much record keeping to do, I wonder if they have any time to actually look after their patients.

The nurses certainly don't have time for family members. I feel scared to ask questions, but am determined to do so anyway. Mom is so scared she just stands there like a statue, and when her time is up and the nurses tell her to leave it is almost like she wants to run away.

Raza is of course treated differently. They seem very keen to answer questions he might have.

He just keeps staring at all the gadgets and asking about them.

The ventilator is the most scary gadget of all. I think if ever needed one, I would rather die. Every now and then the nurse has to shove a suction tube down into Abba-jaan's chest and suck out the sputum. The first time I saw them do it, I thought he was having a convulsion. He even tried to open his eyes and was trying to move his hands.

I asked the nurse why he is so fast asleep and how long do they normally sleep after an operation. She said, Oh he will wake up if we don't keep him sedated. She showed me the pumps that are pumping in the medicines. There are 4 of them stacked one on top of the other on a metal pole (iv stand??). Two are to keep him sedated, and two are to keep his blood pressure steady.

Every hour they turn him. When I went in the morning he was facing one wall, and in the evening he was facing the other. Mom wanted to find out which side is west, so we know when he is facing Mecca. I wanted to ask her, how does it matter when he is so sedated he doesn't know what is going on around him. I have to stop arguing with her. I know she is worried about Dad even more than I am, and we have to wait outside the ICU most of the time hoping everything is going OK inside.

Raza's Diary.

The ICU where they have Dad is a pretty cool place. Very high tech. They actually have a monitoring system with cameras that feed into a screen in the main nursing station, and one person constantly is monitoring it so they can keep an eye on everyone in the ICU. I think they should hook it up to the internet, and we could access the camera feed anywhere in the world. That way patients' families could sit at home much more comfortably and see what's going on and not keep harassing them. Just have to have the ID and password protection built in.

There are 8 beds altogether, although only 4 are occupied at this time. Dad is the most serious one, and is directly in front of the main nursing station. The patients off to the sides have had their liver transplants a few days ago and are recovering.

They monitor the fresh transplant patients very intensively. The tubes coming out of him check blood pressure on the right and left sides of his heart, and there is also a monitor that continuously reads out his cardiac output. That's how many liters his heart is pumping out every minute. I googled it and Dad has a cardiac output above the normal range! I thought that may be because he used to be a boxer and all, but the nurse told me that all cirrhosis patients have a high cardiac output. Wow! Who would have thought that the heart would be stronger than normal in some diseases! Mind boggling! I remember Krishnan-uncle saying that patients waiting for a kidney transplant have to worry their heart will become too weak for a transplant because it gets weak on dialysis. And I automatically assumed the same would be the case for people waiting for a liver transplant. But this nurse says that's not true. She seems to know what she is saying.

Learn something new every day...

Anyway, I am glad these ICU nurses looking after Dad all seem to be very efficient.

BTW, Mom says she will tell me what she wants entered in my diary. She doesn't want to keep a separate diary of her own. And even if she did, I doubt she would let any of us ever read it, so I said OK.

Today Mom has nothing to put in the diary. Just that I should write Dad looks well. I hope that means she is happy with the nursing care he is getting. More likely it is the old "shubh-shubh kaho" thing. She wanted to meet with Dr. A, but we could not. She is determined to meet him tomorrow. Hope he gets enough rest before Mom starts nagging him.

Shehnaz's diary

Day #1

Today Dad's eyes are opening. The swelling is down, and I saw him look at me. I am sure he recognized me. He keeps frowning. I know that frown. It's not his angry frown. It means he wants something.

I asked the nurse if she had asked him what he wants, and she said that he is still sedated, so he may not be able to communicate. So in front of her, I started asking Dad whether he is in pain, and what does he want. He kept shaking his head to say No. No pain, no worry, no fear that we have left him alone, nothing.

Then I asked him if he wanted some water, and he immediately nodded, Yes! Imagine, that! He is being sedated with 2 infusions, and he can still ask for water!

It seems you cannot give water to drink while they have a breathing tube in. But the nurse wet his lips and that seemed to calm him down, and he relaxed and closed his eyes after some time.

It seems his kidneys are not doing too good. He is making less urine than they think he should be. Well, if they gave him some water to drink, it might solve all his problems!

I asked about food. Is it OK not to give him any food for 2 days? They say its fine, no problem in "these patients".

*His eyes look yellow to me. But the nurse said that in artificial light the color is not reliable so they depend on his blood tests, and yes the bilirubin level is up. I am sure she had not noticed it till I asked. Have to ask Dr *(I'll just call him * for Asterix) what is going on. Trouble is nobody seems to know when he will come for rounds.*

This whole system is totally disorganized, I think.

Raza's Diary

I spoke with the Critical Medicine doctor today. Very shy chap, and scared to say anything to anyone, but I thought I had seen him somewhere. Turned out he went to premedical college here and I had seen him at an intercollegiate cultural fest. He used to compete in the Malayalam classical section. His name is Bharatan.

He said they are waiting for the Chief of Anesthesia and Critical Care to come for her rounds today, and then they may take out Dad's breathing tube and stop the ventilator. Very confidential-like he told me that he thinks Dad will be able to come off the ventilator. His chest xray is good, but his kidneys are not working that well, so maybe they will wait for the kidneys to pick up before taking him off the ventilator. Don't know what the connection is, but it seems if they have to start him on dialysis, then its better they start while he is still sedated, so he is more comfortable.

Looked up ventilators on the internet. It's just a glorified pump with a bunch of controls, and gauges to monitor the inflow and outflow etc. Pretty simple concept, actually, but the ventilators they have here cost more than a car! It seems they import all the ventilators, and nobody seems to know why. Maybe it is something to do with licensing of medical devices and products. Easier to get something readymade than to develop it here ourselves.

Mom and Shehnaz are pretty upset at the way the nurses are looking after Dad. I don't really understand, but they have asked for a meeting with Dr. A tomorrow.

Shehnaz's diary

Today is post op Day#3.

I did not write anything in my diary yesterday. There was so much going on that at the end of the day I was exhausted and just went to sleep.

Looks like Dad's new liver is not working properly. The yellow color I had noticed, got worse. Even his nurse stopped trying to tell me it is normal.

In the night they started him on dialysis. They are saying that it is just to support his kidneys, and not because they think the kidneys are not going to work. The dialysis is continuous. Now there is a dialysis nurse always there in addition to his regular nurse. This dialysis nurse doesn't talk at all. Just stands there looking grim (I can only see her eyes above her face mask). They had to put in a dialysis catheter in his groin. That must have been so painful. Guess that is why they kept him sedated.

Finally this afternoon we got to see Dr *. He met with all of us in the side room of the ICU. He said Dad's new liver is not working as well as he likes to see. It is getting his blood acid levels down, and his blood clotting seems to be OK, but the liver function tests are all deranged. There is a liver enzyme which tells him that liver cells are dying, and this test is getting worse.

They do ultrasound scans every day. Dr* says they all show the liver looks OK. The blood flow into it is good, the artery is normal and surgically everything is OK.

But it is not working.

Don't know what will happen. Mother has gone to the mosque to offer special prayers. Mustafa took her, and I told him to take her home first so she could get some clothes for me. I think if I wear the dress Dad gave me for my last birthday it will make him happy. He is more awake now, and smiles at us and raises his hand to reassure us he is OK. Poor chap. He has no idea how bad things are looking. That's good. All I need to do is to somehow keep him happy.

He says he has no pain. How is that even possible? His incision is HUGE. They are calling it a Mercedes Benz incision because it is shaped like that sign in front of the car. How disrespectful!

I don't like the way these doctors and nurses talk about their patients. Comparing them to cars is not respectful. I never want to even see another Mercedes car. I hate German cars anyway.

Raza's diary

Lots of stuff happening. Dad is going high tech. His ventilator is now on a reduced mode, so it kicks in only when he sleeps or if he gets tired. He seems to be more awake, but it is hard to tell. Drifting in and out, his nurse said.

He has dialysis going on continuously. This is a crazy machine with tubes that suck out the blood and send it through a filter. You can see the filter full of blood, and the pump turning, and the blood moving outside the body. The tubes are made of clear plastic. While I was there the filter they were using got clotted and had to be changed. I saw them fill up a new circuit with the dialysis solution which runs on one side of the filter. Then they hooked up the tubes to a catheter they've put in Dad's thigh. And when they started the pump the blood slowly came out and filled the tubes and then flowed into the filter which looks like a cylindrical oil filter that you can put in a car. Only, it is longer. Totally freaky.

I asked Dad how he is doing. He gave me a thumbs up! He's having fun! He is one tough dude!

Can't understand why Dr. A is so full of gloom and doom. I felt like telling him to chill, Dad's going to be fine. It seems some numbers are going up when they do his blood tests. I asked my buddy Bharatan, and he says he has seen this happen before, and the numbers can go so high they go off the scale and the lab does not even report them. Dad is only in the 6000 range, he said. Seems Dr. A gets all uptight if the numbers go over 600.

Dr. A told me that if the numbers don't start coming down, then they may have to re-transplant him. So I asked him if he would use my liver, and he said yes. So I may end up donating my liver to Dad. No problem. I'm cool with that. It's what I told them to do in the first place!

But I won't be telling Mom and Sis about this now. That will totally freak them out.

The ICU nurse, the cute one (her name is Shobha) drew my blood for tests. Hardly felt the needle, but she drew like 10 tubes of blood!

I am writing this as I wait for an MRI scan. They will do the scan only if my blood tests come out normal and OK for me to donate my liver.

Shehnaz's diary

Raza is driving me crazy. He knows something he is not telling me or Mom. I know it. I can see it in his eyes. I tried to look at his diary, but he won't let me read it. I told him he can read mine. I have no secrets. But he refuses. So I am not talking to him now.

I went for breakfast to the cafeteria alone. Mom had gone home early to have a proper shower. She hates the hospital shower. Raza said he was not coming because I keep fighting with him. If Mom finds out he sent me alone to the cafeteria he will get it good from her. Serves him right.

Mom is worried as usual. I keep sending her on errands, so she will be occupied. The more fuss I make the better for her, I think.

Dad is still on the ventilator. I asked the nurses how long they keep people on the ventilator, and they say this is quite normal. It sounded like they are being evasive or giving me a brush-off.

There is some new medicine they are giving Dad. Everyone is quite excited about it, and frankly I don't think they know much about the medicine. They had to get a nurse from the Kidney transplant ICU to come and help them mix it up and give it.

Dr* said that by tonight he will know if this liver is going to work or not. He said he is hopeful because the donor's heart at the Heart Center is working well. The kidney they transplanted in this hospital is working well, he said, but it was slow to start off. Now this liver may be doing something similar, but the difference is that they don't have a way to support it as well as other organs.

What happens if it does not work?

I don't want to know.

I met Mrs. Krishnan in the cafeteria. She saw me sitting alone, and came and sat with me. She is much more friendly now. She said that Mr. Krishnan's new kidney did not work for 1 full day, then slowly picked up. But he is still not doing OK. He had to have dialysis as well, immediately after his transplant got done. It seems his potassium level in the blood had gone too high.

I told her Dad's liver is also not working. She asked me if it was OK with me if she prays for Dad in the temple. I said that's fine with us. I told her Dad always says God listens to everyone, then He does what is right for everyone. He says he learned that during his boxing days.

I told her, what a coincidence! Dad and Krishnan uncle both needing dialysis after their transplant!

Then Mrs. Krishnan said the strangest thing. She said Dad and Krishnan uncle are brothers now, because they have organs from the same donor.

That is so biologically complicated!

In fact it is so complicated on so many levels, I wanted to tell her, Dude, I don't even want to think about it right now. I am just hoping Dad will survive this operation.

Anyway, they have started feeding Dad through a tube. Must be because I kept pestering them. I've realized that they won't do anything unless you keep asking. Now they are worried about Dad's abdomen getting distended, but I have been watching every time they let me in to see him, and nothing like that is happening. I don't want to get blamed for whatever is going wrong, just because I asked them to feed him!

Raza's diary

Got my MRI scan. Man, what a horrible experience! I never want to have another scan. It's like being stuck in a torpedo tube in a submarine! And noisy as hell!

Blood tests all came back good. They checked my EKG and did my heart echo. All good. I can donate if needed. Am on 'liquid diet only' for now. The operation may happen tonight.

Long discussion today with Dr. A and his team. They showed me Dad's flow sheets and charts.

Dad's liver test numbers are nowhere near normal, but there may be some improvement. Won't know for sure till evening.

Dr. A seemed to have a lot of time today. No rush. He said he has a light schedule today … unless he has to take out my liver. That would ruin his evening, he said. He's quite funny.

They showed me all of Dad's charts. I am being treated like a member of the team!

Their charting system is quite obsolete, and is still on paper. They only write progress notes in their electronic medical records. What a waste! The lab inputs the results in the computer, but they have their own format. The doctors and nurses need to see some, but not all of the labs in the form of a spreadsheet. It is so simple to have the labs results automatically populate the spreadsheet, but they say they don't have the software for it. How dumb is that?!

He explained a lot of stuff to me. The spreadsheet runs for 4 weeks at a time, and is arranged in three sections. In one they input all the lab results manually. In another section they enter the results of special tests and culture results to see if there is an infection going on. Then they have the medicines section. They have to keep track of all the medicines, and every day they make a decision about the anti-rejection medicines – which ones to give and what doses. It often takes them a week to ten days to get these rejection medicines right. It's the most tricky part. Everyone is different, and the medicines needed by the immune system are different for each person. Dr. A said that they have to look at everything on the spreadsheet every day before deciding the immunosuppression medicines. He said that is what he gets paid the big bucks to do. Ha ha!

Anyway, he told me that this practice of keeping a chart or a checklist for transplant patients is being done worldwide. This practice is based on solid data that show that having a checklist increases safety and efficiency. They use checklists now for all sorts of complex things – flying planes, constructing skyscrapers, and even for investment banking. He said something very interesting which I think will be good for any business management student: "the management of complexity does not require intelligence. It requires careful attention to detail." And that is what the checklist does.

Dr. A said today he felt like he was taking "Teaching Rounds" like he used to when he was in a teaching hospital. He recommended a book for me: "The Checklist Manifesto" by Atul Gawande. I've heard of it before. It seems Gawande is a surgeon!

I'm already thinking of a dozen different ways in which I can improve stuff just by using checklists properly. Must tell Dad about this. He can sure use this in his business! He is still resisting computers, but a paper checklist is something he will agree to, I am sure. Then whenever I come home from college, I can quickly catch up with everything that is going on, and have some meaningful discussions with him and his staff. Right now it is such a hassle and waste of time trying to figure out what has been going on in the business.

Anyway, if all goes well, then Dad will come off the ventilator by this evening. If not, then we have to do a retransplant using my liver. It will probably be sometime tonight.

Shehnaz is not talking to me today. Thank God. So I did not have to explain any of this to her. When Mom came back she didn't say she went to the cafeteria alone, so Mom just assumed I had gone with her. Thank God again!

Late that evening, Dr. A called the Aliyar Kunju family into the ICU. The day shift was over, and night nurses had come on duty. The hospital as a whole was quiet after the bustle of a busy day. Only the ICU continued as always. It made no difference there if it was day or night.

For the first time the whole family were inside the ICU together, instead of coming one-by-one which was the usual rule. Also, for the first time, they saw Kunju without his breathing tube, and awake. He smiled at them, and reached out to hold each one by the hand. Shehnaz did not let go of his hand through the rest of the visit, standing close by his bed.

The crisis was over, Dr. A informed them. The liver had been slow to start working, and for a while they though he is at risk for "Primary Non-function". This usually means the liver has to be re-transplanted. But that would not be required. Also, dialysis would probably be stopped within 24 hours. He would soon come off all the infusion pumps, and they would be ready to move him out of the ICU in a couple of days.

Already heart, lungs, and kidneys were doing well. When the liver works, everything else settles down fast.

What happened? Don't really know Dr. A said. It is often hard to tell why organs don't work. The only course is to keep checking that all the 'plumbing' is right, and wait and hope for the best.

Ayesha clasped her hands together and looked to heaven, silently breathing a Thank you God prayer.

Shehnaz was not in such a thankful mood. She was not going to let Dr. A off so lightly.

"And what would you have done if it had not worked?" she asked edgily.

"Your brother. Ask him. He was going to donate his liver. The work up was completed this morning."

Both Shehnaz and Ayesha stared at Raza open-mouthed, in shock. Kunju reached out for his son with his free hand, and held him tight.

"But you never told us!" mother and daughter said in unison. It was not clear whether they were addressing Raza, or Dr. A, or both.

"That was Raza's decision. He did not want us to tell you. He said he would tell you himself in due course. Legally he is old enough, and he can give consent himself. We cannot involve any family members in his decision unless he gives us permission to do so. But now, since the need will not arise, I have taken the liberty to tell you what his decision was."

"You mean you can take out his liver without asking his mother?" Ayesha asked indignantly.

"Yes Ma'am. Legally, I can. Unfortunately there are people who do this all the time – donate organs without informing their family members. I would probably not have taken your son to the Operation Theater unless you were also informed. But your objections would not have taken priority over his consent. Well, here is the Consent Form he signed. You can tear it up, or keep it as a souvenir."

"I think I will keep it," said Ayesha looking sternly at her son, "and you! You will put this in *my* diary!"

Two weeks later Mohammed Aliyar Kunju was discharged from hospital to home. Mustafa picked the best time to leave the hospital when traffic was at the minimum. He then proceeded to drive so carefully and so slowly, that cars and even scooters began honking at them and overtaking. With masterly self-restraint, Mustafa resisted their enticements to honk back and show them some speed.

At home the guest bedroom downstairs had been fixed up for Kunju. A full couch had been moved in for family members who would be taking turns to stay with him round the clock. A tray table at his bedside would be where he could eat if he did not feel up to going to the dining room. A new TV had been mounted on the wall which he would face when propped up in bed, and the VCR was connected. Raza had a exercise video playing for Kunju as he entered.

"That's what you are going to be doing in one month from now, Dad! So start learning the moves! Meanwhile ...."

He had a surprise gift for his father: a Hi Def collection of Mohammed Ali's fights, and the entire series of Rocky and Rambo movies.

About a month later, Ayesha and Shehnaz set out with Mustafa driving, to go to the hospital where Kunju's donor had been admitted. They had called ahead, and Sunita was waiting for them. From the hospital, they proceeded to Jose Avirachen's house. It was evening, and Sunita would be dropped off at her house afterwards as she had finished work for the day. Sunita had chosen this time as she knew Priya would be back from school. She particularly wanted the two women to meet Priya.

Seleena, Jose Avirachen's widow, had agreed very reluctantly to meet with the family of a recipient. Sunita had to call several times, and spend a long time on the phone with her before she finally agreed.

After Jose's death, Seleena had lost all interest in keeping her house spruced up as she had always done. The garden was not tended, and the flower pots had a profusion of weeds growing out of them. The drawing room had newspapers piled up on the coffee table, and the couch had pencil and ink stains where the children did their homework. She did not mind that they were not willing to go to their room and study. It was nice to have them around her as she sat every evening wondering what to do with her time.

Jose's parents rarely visited. When they did, there was a tension in the air. She wished she had died, and Jose had been here in her place. They would have been all the help he needed, she was certain. The children would soon have forgotten her and moved on with their lives.

There was a picture of Jose on the mantel, above the fake fireplace. The indoor plants in flower pots at the base were among the few things she tended to these days. The only other attempt at decoration, on another shelf, was a garish picture of Jesus wearing bright blue, and his bleeding heart bright red. Her mother-in-law had wanted both pictures placed together. It was yet another thing they disagreed on. If only Jose had told everyone where he wanted his picture, Seleena thought angrily, there would have been no need for any argument or unpleasantness.

She was trying to collect Jose's life insurance. The insurance company and its agents who were all over them when they were shopping for insurance, were now playing hide-and-seek with her. She had known this would happen, but she had not anticipated how low would be her will power when dealing with them. There was something cheap about her trying to collect the money. And truth be told, she did not want it. Once she collected, it would mark another end point in her life and Jose's life. She did not want to drag things on, but she did not want The End either.

Mustafa turned the car into the driveway slowing down to a crawl. On either side moss covered walls of *'vettu-kall'* hemmed the driveway with barely enough space to squeeze through. The engine slowed down to a whisper and with only the sound of tires crunching on gravel they turned into the courtyard of the modest house where Kunju's liver donor had once lived.

Again, Ayesha found herself thinking this might not be a good idea. What if the lady they had come to meet was angry or abusive? What if she asked for too much money? How much was too much? Kunju had given clear instructions. Find out what she wants, multiply by 3, and promise it will be given. They would honor his principle that he would owe no man anything.

"It's all very well to say you will owe no man anything," Ayesha had argued, "but how can anyone put a price on what you, and we, have received?"

"OK. Just go and talk and get an idea of what they want or need, or would like to have. We will discuss it when you get back," replied Kunju, thinking that if only there were a man in that house he would have gone himself and done the deal.

The house was silent, and looked deserted. The garden was a mess. Shehnaz had her iPad with her, and took a couple of pictures.

Sunita strode confidently to the door and rang the bell. She was the only one among the three women who was comfortable in these surroundings. Also, she had been here before.

Soon the door opened, and Seleena stood framed in the doorway. A little boy stood beside her, clinging to her sari. She smiled quickly at Sunita, then looked searchingly at the two women. After what seemed like eternity, she invited them in.

The drawing room had been cleaned up, but the cushion covers on the sofa were crumpled, and looked like they had seen better days. The carpet covering the red oxide floor did not match the cushions, and both ends were curling, as though the carpet had been recently unrolled from storage.

They sat in the circle fixed by the furniture, keeping their feet off the carpet. Sunita reached over to try and play with the little boy who Seleena had kept clutched in her lap. It was not clear who was clinging to whom.

Chaffing at the restraint, the boy wriggled free, jumped to the floor and seated himself cross-legged on the carpet. Looking at his visitors he said solemnly, "This is a new carpet. Mom had kept it rolled up. We got it for everyone to sit on when they came to see my Daddy's coffin."

"Really?" said Sunita, hoping this conversational topic would change, but succeeding only in prolonging it.

"Yes, they sang songs all night. So many songs!" gesturing with his arms widespread, "I fell asleep right here on the carpet."

"Oh, he is so cute!" Sunita gushed, her face crumpling.

"I look like my Daddy," the little boy said, continuing in his serious tone. "See, that's his picture there. Mommy said that Jesus picture should be on the other shelf. There. Grandma said …"

"OK son, that is enough," interrupted Seleena sternly. "You need to be quiet when we have guests, or I will send you to your room."

Chided, the little boy fell silent, focusing his attention on Shehnaz who he seemed to find most interesting.

"Where is my friend Priya?" asked Sunita.

"She will be here soon. Her school bus should come any moment now. Can I get you all some coffee?

Ayesha said no, thank you. Sunita said yes, and recognizing the real reason for the offer, Shehnaz said yes as well. Seleena picked up her son and escaped through the doorway to the back of the house, leaving her visitors alone in the drawing room.

They spoke in hushed whispers, Ayesha asking Sunita if she would introduce the topic as to how they could help the family. She whispered back that she felt very uncomfortable talking about a financial compensation, but she would find out what the needs were, and get back to them later. For now it was sufficient that they meet and get to know each other, and they should probably leave after they had coffee.

Just then, with a pounding of running feet on the gravel outside, and a crash, the front door was thrown open. A skinny girl wide eyed and breathless in pig-tails and a blue pinafore school uniform, lugging a school bag that seemed twice her weight, stood framed in the doorway. She bit her lower lip as she looked from one guest to the other, her mouth twisting into a hesitant smile, and then into a big grin when she saw Sunita.

"Hullo Priya!" Sunita jumped up with a little gasp, "just look at you. You've grown taller in just one month since I saw you! Come here, let me give you a big hug!"

There was a definite change in the girl she knew. She was thinner, and probably taller, but the sudden growth was not entirely a physical change. There was something on a deeper plane that had matured in the girl Sunita knew.

Shehnaz had also stood up, involuntarily, as she gazed at the girl who was responsible for giving her father a new life. The elfin face, huge bright eyes and the incandescent smile had her goggling in admiration at the little girl half her age. She wanted to hug her, just instantly in love with this new person in her life. New, yes, but constantly on her mind, ever since she heard from Sunita the story of how Priya had initiated the organ donation when her father died. She was everything she had imagined. She was more than everything.

"Hello Priya," Shehnaz said, suddenly shy, embarrassed at the flood of emotion, "I am Shehnaz."

Priya broke free from Sunita's embrace, and met Shehnaz's wide eyed stare with a matching gaze of her own.

"Can I really call you Shehnaz?" she asked, her face dimpling with a mixture of happiness and doubt that she could take such liberties.

"Of course!" said Shehnaz kneeling down to bring her face on the same level as the little girl, "or if you want you can call me 'Didi'. I always imagined having a little sister just like you!"

Artlessly Priya embraced her. Shehnaz barely able to control her tears, could not stop a sniffle.

"And this is your Aunty Ayesha," said Shehnaz introducing her mother.

"Hullo Priya," Ayesha said more formally, and asked the inevitable question Malayalis ask little children, "what class are you in?"

"I am in standard 6 B," Priya said in her best sing-song classroom voice, enunciating each word clearly.

Ayesha's attempt at being formal dissolved, as she shook her head in wonder at how such a simple answer could also be so endearing.

"Come here, darling. Let me also give you a hug."

Priya stepped forward instantly, dutifully, without a trace of shyness, to accept the embrace, standing straight as Ayesha buried her face in the little shoulder.

The visitors were shamelessly teary and choking, as Seleena brought in a tray with three cups of coffee.

The visit, which Ayesha had planned would be short, stretched to over an hour. The little boy who had greeted them when they arrived had gotten bored with them, and was fast asleep in his mother's lap. Shehnaz and Priya, who had bonded right away, sat curled up together, feet on the sofa, as Shehnaz showed the younger girl her iPad, and all the different wonders it performed. They took pictures of everyone and shot selfies as well, laughing happily at how ridiculous they looked at arm's length. Priya dragged her schoolbag to the floor below the sofa, and together they proceeded to do Internet searches on Priya's homework assignments, cleaning up each task rapidly, as Priya squealed with happiness at how wonderfully the work was going!.

Seleena sat with the older women speaking little. She enquired how Kunju was doing, and smiled wistfully when told he was well. She listened with interest as Ayesha described how she had to manage his medicines, and how he had started trying to lose weight. How much energy he now had! And he and Raza were full of plans, discussing all kinds of things related to work. Raza had decided he was going to join his father in business. He used to have no interest in it, and would talk of all sorts of other things he wanted to do, and travel etc., but now it looked like he had made up his mind. They were like brothers now, not father and son any more.

Sunita finally broached the subject of what they could do for Seleena. The enquiry did not go well. Seleena buried her face in her hands, and sobbed quietly. Priya looked up from the cooperative homework exercise, stared at her mother quietly for a moment, and then at Sunita and Ayesha who were looking embarrassed. She crinkled her eyes, and motioned reassuringly with her hand signaling "She will be OK, don't worry. I'll take care of it later."

After a while, when they were ready to leave, Shehnaz asked Seleena, "Is it OK if I get Priya a laptop computer and an internet connection? She learns so fast! She's already learned how to access the internet. She says there are kids in her class who have their own computers. I want to come back this weekend and fix up an email account for her. Maybe get her on Facebook as well! That is how I can stay in touch with her when I leave for college. We can chat every day! There's tons of stuff we can do together!"

"Please Mom, say yes, Mom," urged Priya, as Seleena looked doubtful.

"Jose used to say he was going to get her a computer, but ..." her voice trailed off.

"OK. Let's do it like this. I will come back this weekend and bring the computer, and then you can decide. OK?" said Shehnaz, in her most business-like voice.

"Say OK, Mom. Say OK!"

"OK," said Seleena, her voice barely above a whisper. "Thank you all for coming. It has meant so much for me. For all of us. I feel stronger now. We are going to be alright. Don't worry about us. Give your husband my regards. And also your son."

And with that they said their goodbyes and left.

On the way to Sunita's house, they discussed what Sunita knew about Jose Avirachen's family.

He had married Seleena without the complete approval of his parents. Something about her dowry. Their main income was from running the two shops that had been the family business. After the accident, Jose's parents claimed absolute rights to these properties, and had explicitly denied Seleena any share in the proceeds if they were sold, as they almost certainly would be, after the dust settled. Seleena could assert her rights and run the shops, perhaps, but the daily commute from their house to the business was not something she wanted to do, especially after Jose killed himself doing it. Right now, her priorities were the children and looking after them.

"Is there no support from her own family?" asked Ayesha. She was thinking of Muslim personal law which says a woman should be looked after by her father and brothers if her marriage fell apart.

"There is a brother in Dubai, but he is married and has a family of his own."

"Yes, we know how that goes. Just wait for the oil prices or the exchange rate to drop and his interest in his sister will be secondary to his interest in his savings," said Ayesha gloomily.

After dropping Sunita off at her home, they drove back hurriedly as it was time for Kunju's evening medication, and Ayesha wanted to be sure she was there when he took his pills. The dose of one of his immunosuppression medications had been changed at the last clinic visit, and she wanted to be sure he got it right.

Kunju and Raza were eager to hear how the visit with their donor's family had gone. Shehnaz did most of the talking as they had dinner, reaching out with one hand to show them all the pictures she had taken on her iPad.

"Dad, I've promised Priya I will get her a computer. Is that OK?"

"Certainly, my dear. I am glad you have decided to keep in contact with the girl. Whatever help she needs we will do our best. You only have to say the word."

Raza and Shehnaz immediately began arguing over which was the best computer to buy. A short list was generated, and the trip to the store was planned.

"That's all very well," said Raza, returning to the original discussion "but what about the mother. Don't you want to give her some cash to help them manage? They sound like they could use it."

Like his father, he too had an aversion to the feeling of being in debt to anyone.

"Yes. Absolutely. They must be having financial needs, and we have to help them financially," Kunju was quick to agree, "Ayesha, have you thought of an amount?"

Ayesha had been silent most of the evening, busy with serving dinner. She had hardly eaten anything herself. Brimming emotions from earlier in the evening had left her with no interest in food. She sat now, facing her family, all that she held most precious, and spoke from her heart.

"You know, when we were at that house, I was reminded of the house we lived in when you kids were that age. It was not much different from that. At that time we too had financial needs. So many! I thought about money all the time! I remember once we asked the bank for a loan, and the interest rate was so high, almost twenty per cent! We could never have paid that much. So we decided to approach one of Dad's uncles for a loan, and he flatly refused to help. It was so humiliating! But that experience made us more determined to succeed. We managed with less, and we took very careful financial decisions, and always repaid the loans we took. Never owe anything, was our motto, and it helped us make good decisions."

"Yes," Kunju said, smiling at the recollection. "That uncle was a character! His son now owes us, and there is no mention of repayment! But your mother was the one who stretched each penny we had. I still don't know how your school expenses, and uniforms and fees, and everything else got paid for with the miserable salary I brought home to her at the beginning of each month. You kids and I never went hungry, though there were nights, like tonight, when I did not see your mother eat dinner."

Raza and Shehnaz loved to hear such stories. Their parents rarely talked to them about the tough times they had faced together.

Ayesha continued.

"So I think a lump sum of money now is not the right thing for Seleena. She needs a job. She said she is prepared to take anything that will give her time to spend with the kids. I will talk to Mrs. Krishnan. She was saying her brother works for a Bank, and I read in the paper it is opening a new branch in that area. That may be a good job, with benefits and enough time to manage the home and the kids, and avenues for promotion as well. If that doesn't work out we have other friends we can influence to find her a job.

"What I plan to do is to open an educational trust account for both the kids to pay for their school and college education. We can link it to an insurance policy that starting right now will cover their medical needs right through to the time they finish college. Paying for our health care and your education as kids, used to worry me the most when I was Seleena's age. With that worry out of the way, Seleena's job and salary will give her the independence and motivation she needs to succeed on her own."

"And I will be in touch with Priya anyway, so if anything unusual pops up we can step in at that time," added Shehnaz.

"We can also ask Sunita to let us know if any sudden expenses arise. She had said she is going to keep in touch with Seleena on a regular basis, and anyway the hospital she works at is where they will probably go for all their needs."

Kunju listened to the plans approvingly. He had never thought he would see a day when a debt he could never repay would actually make him happy.

THE END

Appendix 1

Glasgow Coma Score

The GCS is scored between 3 and 15, 3 being the worst, and 15 the best. It is composed of three parameters: Best Eye Response, Best Verbal Response, Best Motor Response, as given below:

Best Eye Response. (4)

1. No eye opening.
2. Eye opening to pain.
3. Eye opening to verbal command.
4. Eyes open spontaneously.

Best Verbal Response. (5)

1. No verbal response
2. Incomprehensible sounds.
3. Inappropriate words.
4. Confused
5. Orientated

Best Motor Response. (6)

1. No motor response.
2. Extension to pain.
3. Flexion to pain.
4. Withdrawal from pain.
5. Localising pain.
6. Obeys Commands.

Note that the phrase 'GCS of 11' is essentially meaningless, and it is important to break the figure down into its components, such as E3V3M5 = GCS 11.

A Coma Score of 13 or higher correlates with a mild brain injury, 9 to 12 is a moderate injury and 8 or less a severe brain injury.

Teasdale G., Jennett B., LANCET (ii) 81-83, 1974.

Appendix 2

Upanishad quotation

(extracted from 'The Principal Upanishads – a poetic transcreation' by Alan Jacobs.)

Yagnavalkya said,

When that Self has sunk into death

It sinks into unconsciousness

Then gathers the senses

Around him or her,

And gathering the elements of light

Falls into the Heart.

When the supreme in the eye turns away

It ceases to recognize any names or forms.

He or she has become One

With the Self as Brahman.

He or she does not see

Smell,

Taste,

Speak,

Hear,

Think,

Touch,

Know.

The heart center is lit up

By 'That', Consciousness, which leaves

Through the eye or skull

When his or her knowledge and deeds

Take him or her to the world of Brahman.

The life breath leaves

With all other vital forces.

APPENDIX 3

HEALTH AND FAMILY WELFARE (S) DEPARTMENT
G.O (MS)No.37/2012/H&FWD Dated,
Thiruvananthapuram, 04.02.2012
Read: - G.O.(MS)No.36/2012/H&FWD dated 04.02.2012

ORDER

4. One of the major impediments in deceased donor transplantation in the State is the lack of clarity in brain death certification and its optional nature. There are also doubts in medical circles on the authority by which doctors may declare "Brain Death", whenever required. *The Transplantation of Human Organs Act, 1994 (THOA, 1994) and the Transplantation of Human Organs Rules, 1995 (THO Rules) made there under are the only pieces of legislation available wherein brain death certification procedures have been elaborately laid down, it is hereby decided that the procedures outlined therein will also be adopted as brain death certification procedure in Kerala. This order will also elaborate on the above format to ensure its applicability to the entire State of Kerala. Government therefore hereby order and made it mandatory that whenever the medical condition (clinical and medical criteria have been met for) of a patient has reached a brain death stage, brain death certification is done as stipulated in this order.* This will come into force

with immediate effect in all Government District Hospitals & General Hospitals and all the 5 Government Medical Colleges and Private hospitals in the State registered as Transplant Centres with the Appropriate Authority for certifying Brain Death as per the THO Act, in the event of a family of brain dead person consenting to organ donation. All Organ Transplantation Centres will register with the Appropriate Authority for this purpose.

ACKNOWLEDGMENTS

Getting a manuscript to publication is to experience a complex and intimidating world. Having not done anything more difficult than surgery and publishing articles in scientific journals, I needed a lot of help. My daughter, Ranjana Collins, in Austin, Texas, brought her media production skills to the task, rolling away every obstacle and finding the best people to help me. She has been my guide, mentor, and encouragement, and has produced this book.

Adam Gardner edited Transplant Story. He soon realized, I think, that special persuasive skills are required to make edits when dealing with a cantankerous surgeon who regarded every written line as a step in an operation note. He has deep understanding of different styles of English and appreciated and preserved my Indian 'accents' while ironing out convolutions that creep into my prose from other languages employed by me and the characters in this story.

Courtney Andujar designed the book cover. A dark night sky turning to dawn is her apt pictorial interpretation of transplantation. In the trees filtering the light of a new day, you can recognize the coconut palms that are typical of Kerala in India where the story is located.

My good friend and venerable senior from medical school, Professor G.M. Siddiqui—currently Head of the Anatomy department at MOSC Medical College in Kolenchery, is the creator of the illustrations in this book. A natural artist, who illustrates his lectures drawing freehand on a blackboard, he took my sketches and gave them the professional touch they needed for publication.

In this book I have tried to interest the reader in different aspects of organ transplant. However, each case is unique as an individual donor heals individual recipients, and those who witness this miracle unfold may have experiences, ideas and questions of their own. The best compliment that I can hope for is that Transplant Story creates an ongoing channel of communication between my readers and me. If you have specific questions or opinions to share, please visit www.organtransplantinformation.com.

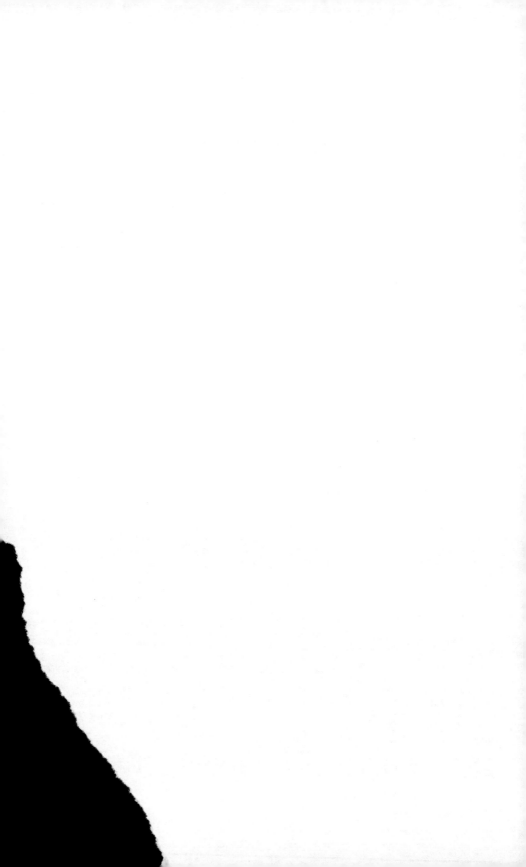

Printed in the United States
By Bookmasters